An Atlas of
ONCOLOGY

THE ENCYCLOPEDIA OF VISUAL MEDICINE SERIES

An Atlas of
ONCOLOGY

Ronald W. Raven

O.B.E.(Mil.), O.St.J., T.D., F.R.C.S., Hon. F.R.S.M.

With a special foreword by R. Begent,
The Ronald Raven Professor of Oncology,
The Royal Free Hospital, London

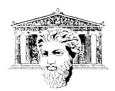

The Parthenon Publishing Group
International Publishers in Medicine, Science & Technology

Casterton Hall, Carnforth,
Lancs, LA6 2LA, UK

One Blue Hill Plaza, Pearl River,
New York 10965, USA

Ronald W. Raven was formerly:

Consulting Surgeon, Royal Marsden Hospital and Institute of Cancer Research

Consulting Surgeon, Westminster Hospital

Member, Court of Patrons (late Council); Erasmus Wilson Lecturer; Arris and Gale Lecturer; Bradshaw Lecturer; and Hunterian Professor, The Royal College of Surgeons of England

Founder President, British Association of Surgical Oncology. Founder President, Head and Neck Oncologists of Great Britain

President Marie Curie Memorial Foundation

President Epsom College

British Library Cataloguing-in-Publication Data
Raven, Ronald W.
    Atlas of Oncology. – (Encyclopedia of Visual Medicine series)
    I. Title   II. Series
    616.99
    ISBN 1-85070-363-9

Library of Congress Cataloging-in-Publication Data
Raven, Ronald William.
    An atlas of oncology/ Ronald W. Raven
        p.   cm. – (The Encyclopedia of visual medicine series)
    Includes bibliographical references and index.
    ISBN 1-86070-363-9
    I. Cancer–Atlases.   2. Cancer–Histopathology–Atlases.
I. Title.   II. Series.
[DNLM: I. Neoplasms–atlases. QZ 17 R253a]

RC 262.R39   1992
616.99'4–dc20
DNLM/DLC
for Library of Congress   92-49121
                                                            CIP

Published in the UK and Europe by
The Parthenon Publishing Group Limited
Casterton Hall, Carnforth
Lancs. LA6 2LA

Published in North America by
The Parthenon Publishing Group Inc.
One Blue Hill Plaza
PO Box 1564, Pearl River
New York 10965, USA

Copyright © 1994 Parthenon Publishing Group Ltd

First published 1994

Typeset by AMA Graphics Ltd., Preston
Printed and bound in Spain by T.G. Hostench, S.A.

Contents

The Encyclopedia of Visual Medicine Series

Titles currently planned in this series include:

An Atlas of Oncology
An Atlas of Hypertension
An Atlas of Common Diseases
An Atlas of Osteoporosis
An Atlas of the Menopause
An Atlas of Contraception
An Atlas of Endometriosis
An Atlas of Ultrasonography in Obstetrics and Gynecology
An Atlas of Practical Radiology
An Atlas of Psoriasis
An Atlas of Trauma Management
An Atlas of Lung Infections
An Atlas of Transvaginal Color Doppler
An Atlas of Child Health
An Atlas of Infective Endocarditis
An Atlas of Rheumatology
An Atlas of Epilepsy
An Atlas of HIV and AIDS-related Diseases
An Atlas of Practical Dermatology
An Atlas of Laser Operative Laparoscopy and Hysteroscopy
An Atlas of Atherosclerosis
An Atlas of Eye Diseases
An Atlas of Cutaneous Growths
An Atlas of Myocardial Infarction

Series Foreword

The art of effective diagnosis is one that relies to a considerable degree – although certainly not exclusively – on the recognition of visual signs and manifestations of disease. The objective of the Series is to provide a practical aid to diagnosis by illustrating and explaining the wide range of visual signs that a physician needs to be aware of in current medical practice.

Whilst the visual manifestations of disease themselves remain constant, the development of new techniques of invasive and non-invasive diagnosis means that new images are frequently being added to the range of visual material that the diagnostician must be familiar with: ultrasound, radiology, magnetic resonance imaging, endoscopy and photomicrography all provide examples of this kind of material. It is the intention of this Series to document, where appropriate, the result of such techniques and to explain and elucidate their relevance – in addition to documenting all the more standard visual images.

The Series is also distinctive in that individual volumes will focus on carefully selected, specific topics, which can be covered in some detail – rather than on generalized and broadly-based subject areas that could not easily be covered so thoroughly.

The authors contributing to the Series have all been selected for their special expertise in their own chosen fields, their access to outstanding visual material and their ability to explain the significance of it in an effective and lucid way. Finally, particular emphasis is being placed on achieving a very high quality of colour reproduction in the printing process itself in order to do full justice to the wide variety of visual images presented.

It is hoped that this carefully structured and systematic approach to the visually significant aspects of medicine will make a valuable and ongoing contribution to good diagnostic practice.

Preface

The compilation of an Atlas of Oncology is a task and challenge of considerable magnitude. In accepting this challenge I decided that the contents of the book should be entirely my own work which I have carried out for more than 50 years. During this long period I have seen impressive developments in the prevention, diagnosis and treatment of cancer. A most important advance has now occurred – cancer has become 'oncology'.

The acceleration of scientific knowledge concerning the nature and aetiology of tumours and the extent of their clinical management and treatment have developed so that, from their synthesis, the multidisciplinary subject of oncology has now emerged. This is the vehicle for our scientific knowledge and clinical expertise concerning the multitudinous tumours which for centuries were grouped together indiscriminately under the general term 'cancer'. All the arts and sciences of oncology are now focused upon the nature, causation and management of tumours. The basic sciences continue to make valuable contributions to the theory of oncology whilst the practice of oncology has been developed by clinicians, medical and nursing, and other members of the caring professions.

These tumours occur in nations throughout the world. As a result of epidemiological research we know that their incidence is variable in different countries. They are universally feared because they cause a high mortality rate, considerable morbidity and suffering. Consequently, an international effort is essential to prevent and control these different tumours, and this effort continues to strengthen and expand. We cannot remain complacent, for much work remains to be done.

In the meantime, having regard to the considerable fear, shock and suffering which are engendered in so many people and patients by the word 'cancer', I stress the need to discard this term for all these tumours and substitute oncological diseases and tumours. Following the international establishment and recognition of the term 'oncology', I am convinced it is logical and appropriate to make use of this new nomenclature. The term 'cancer' is now outmoded and has no scientific meaning in the context of disease nomenclature, for it is given to a large number of tumours and diseases with diverse aetiology, manifestation and behaviour which require different forms of research, clinical care and management. The association by this new nomenclature of these tumours and diseases with the master subject of oncology will not only allow these important distinctions, but it also conforms with the nomenclature of other large groups of diseases. Good examples include dermatological diseases associated with dermatology and gynaecological diseases associated with gynaecology.

The number of tumours that develop in the human race is enormous and their significance is very variable. A number are benign and cause no threat to life. Many others are malignant and dangerous, although they vary in their malignant potential; not only do they spread by direct extension to involve contiguous tissues and organs, but dissemination occurs and metastatic tumours are formed in other parts of the body. In my Atlas of Oncology I wish to make it plain that I do not claim to cover the whole extensive spectrum of tumours. I have included in this book only those tumours which have occurred in my own patients. Consequently, the book is a portrayal of my own professional work and experience in the diagnosis, treatment, rehabilitation and continuing care of my own patients over a period of more than 50 years. Important tumours are omitted, as in the lung and uterus, as these require the skill of specialists in these regions.

In the Atlas of Oncology it is clearly apparent how many tumours have changed in their first presentation to clinicians; this is largely due to early diagnosis, so that advanced tumours are becoming increasingly uncommon. An outstanding example of this change is shown by carcinoma of the breast; in fact these advanced tumours of the breast are becoming rare and my illustrations are of much historic interest. The introduction of mammography and ultrasound diagnostic techniques has made a profound change in this dangerous disease.

Personally, I have always found the study of case records of individual patients both helpful and edifying, for so much can be learnt from their symptomatology, diagnosis, treatment and rehabilitation, in addition to their survival. In this book, with the description of various tumours, I have included many of my case records, some in great detail. This gives a clear picture of the clinical effects of these tumours, the treatment which was carried out and the end results. I always keep careful case records of all my patients including clinical photographs taken during various stages of their treatment together with photographs and descriptions of their tumours and the histopathology. I am grateful to my patients, who readily agreed to the taking of the clinical photographs. All these case records have now provided me with all the data I required to write this book.

I wish to express my deepest gratitude to Joan Gough-Thomas, MA for all the splendid help and support she has always given to me in the professional work throughout many years. In particular, she has maintained most efficiently the patients' case record system and has greatly helped in abstracting material for this book. I am very grateful to David Bloomer of the Parthenon Publishing Group for his valuable collaboration in publishing this book. In all my professional work I have been ably supported by splendid colleagues, both senior and junior, and I have greatly enjoyed our work together in helping so many patients. I am full of gratitude to all the members of the nursing profession who have cared for and comforted my patients by day and by night, and for their skilful help in the operation theatres.

The courage of my patients, both young and old and of different nationalities, and their gratitude for help and support for them and their families have been my constant inspiration and encouragement. It has been a real privilege to care for them.

Ronald W. Raven

Foreword

Ronald Raven had an international reputation as a surgeon and oncologist who devoted more than 50 years of his professional life to oncology, including clinical research and prevention of cancer and in the treatment, care and rehabilitation of patients suffering from this disease. His outstanding work was recognized by the many honours bestowed upon him and by his numerous professional appointments. He was Consultant Surgeon to the Royal Marsden Hospital and Institute of Cancer Research, and to the Westminster Hospital where he was Lecturer in Surgery. He was Teacher in Surgery at the University of London and held important lectureships at the Royal College of Surgeons of England where he was Hunterian Professor, Member of Council and Member of the Court of Patrons.

His deep interest in the problems of patients with cancer extended throughout the world. He conducted surgical missions to many countries and lectured world-wide. He was created Chevalier de La Légion d'Honneur and elected a Member of the Academy of Athens. He was Chairman of several International Cancer Associations, Chairman of the Marie Curie Memorial Foundation, Chairman and President of the Royal Medical Foundation of Epsom College, a Fellow of the Royal Society of Medicine and a Freeman of the City of London. He gave distinguished service in the 1939–45 war, being mentioned in despatches and awarded the OBE (Mil.) and later the TD.

Ronald Raven's experiences in the Middle East, Africa, South America and throughout Europe give readers of this book an insight into international variations in incidence and presentation of tumours, which is of particular contemporary value. This Atlas has the authority that only such extensive personal experience as the author's can give.

Author of many standard books on cancer, Ronald Raven kept meticulous records throughout his long career. This book is based on those records and shows how the incidence of cancer has changed over the years, as well as the long-term results of treatment in rare tumour types.

Ronald Raven was a pioneer in the total care of the patient and family. He taught that 'Rehabilitation of patients begins with the diagnosis of cancer' and he had a major influence on modern thinking in this field. He supported the development of oncology nursing and he refined surgical techniques and postoperative care to aid rehabilitation. A ward is named after him in the Rehabilitation Unit which he opened at the Royal Marsden Hospital. He worked tirelessly for the continuing care of people with cancer. In his last years, in addition to writing this and other books, he gave his support, energy and wisdom to establish the 'Ronald Raven Chair in Clinical Oncology' at the Royal Free Hospital School of Medicine, and was able to see it opened by HRH The Princess Royal before he died in October 1991.

R. H. J. Begent
Ronald Raven Professor
Royal Free Hospital School of Medicine
London, UK

1

Tumours of the mouth

THE LIP

Tumours of the lips are relatively uncommon and they are usually squamous cell carcinomas. A basal cell carcinoma has a tendency to occur in the skin of the face but it is rare in the lips. A mixed salivary tumour is rarely seen in this locality and a sarcoma is very rare. A malignant melanoma is also very rare.

Carcinoma

A squamous cell carcinoma may occur in the upper or the lower lip and it is more frequently seen in males than in females. The tumour is becoming increasingly uncommon, which may be associated with the elimination of smoking with a clay pipe. Excessive exposure to sunlight may be a predisposing factor in its development.

Appearance

The lower lip is affected more frequently than the upper lip and the lesion usually appears to one side of the midline. In some patients the angle of the mouth is affected with involvement of the upper and lower lips. An early carcinoma may be a roughened rounded area of thickening of the epidermis, or a flattened bluish-white or grey patch which is difficult to distinguish from leukoplakia. Sometimes there is a fissure or a small ulcer. Later there may be a malignant ulcer, or a nodular or papillomatous tumour (Figure 1).

Histopathology

The tumour presents the same microscopical appearances as a squamous cell carcinoma in the mouth.

Spread of the disease

The carcinoma spreads in the lip by direct extension and gradually destroys the soft tissues in its neighbourhood. Therefore, the angle of the mouth, the skin of the face, and the gingivolabial groove and the alveolus are ultimately affected.

Lymphatic spread occurs to form metastases in the regional lymph nodes. When the carcinoma affects the midline of the lower lip, the submental lymph nodes are affected, and when it is situated more laterally, the submaxillary lymph nodes and later the upper deep cervical lymph nodes become involved. In some patients the carcinoma forms metastases in the pre-auricular lymph nodes.

In carcinoma of the upper lip, metastases may occur in the upper deep cervical lymph nodes and in the pre-auricular and postauricular groups. At first, the lymph nodes are hard in consistency and mobile, but later they become fixed. When the lymph node metastases are extensive, necrosis occurs, cyst-like cavities are produced and the overlying skin becomes

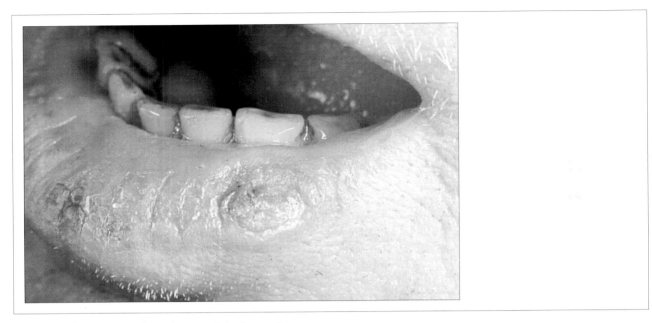

Figure 1 Squamous cell carcinoma of the lower lip

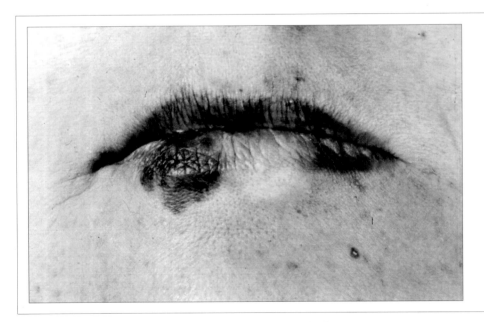

Figure 2 Malignant melanoma of the lower lip which had formed metastases in the left submandibular lymph node

soft and purple; eventually fungation occurs through the skin. Severe haemorrhage occurs if these metastatic lymph nodes invade the internal jugular vein or the carotid arteries.

Spread by the bloodstream is rare so that distant metastases are very infrequent.

Symptoms and signs
These have been clearly described in the preceding sections on the appearance and methods of spread of carcinoma of the lip.

Treatment
A squamous cell carcinoma of the lip is usually treated by a course of radiotherapy. If the tumour is not controlled, surgical excision is carried out. An early small carcinoma can also be treated satisfactorily by a wedge excision and reconstruction of the lip. The regional lymph nodes are treated as for other sites.

Malignant melanoma
A malignant melanoma is a very rare tumour of the lip. Metastases develop in the regional lymph nodes in addition to other sites. The treatment is wide local excision of the primary tumour and excision of metastatic regional lymph nodes. A reconstruction of the lip is carried out.

A patient with a malignant melanoma of the lower lip was referred by another surgeon for an opinion.

Case record A female aged 49 years had developed a swelling in the region of the left submandibular salivary gland which had enlarged rapidly over a period of 5 weeks from the size of a pea to that of a walnut. The surgeon had excised this tumour which was round and encapsulated and separate from the submandibular salivary gland, and which shelled out fairly easily, though in one place the capsule was a little adherent and split during removal. The tumour was soft, almost bluish in colour and partly necrotic. A section showed the appearance of a metastasis of malignant melanoma in a lymph node and a very active tumour. Following this operation and with the histological findings in mind, the surgeon examined very critically, a pigmented area on the right side of her lower lip. The patient stated that this area of pigmentation had commenced on the left side of the lower lip about 3 years previously and had gradually extended across to the right side involving the mucous membrane of the lip and extending for half an inch on the skin. The patient stated that at one period, there had been a tiny ulcer in the midline of the lip almost at the mucocutaneous junction which had left a tiny scar. She had noticed no thickening of the lip but the pigmentation had recently darkened and become tender to extend.

On examination of this patient, no abnormality in the nasopharynx, oropharynx, hypopharynx or larynx was found. The pigmented lesion in the lower lip was not ulcerated, raised from the surface or moist and it showed no clinical evidence of activity (Figure 2). There was some induration around the scar in the left submandibular region and a tiny right submental lymph node was palpable; no other abnormality was felt in the neck.

The further management of this patient was carefully considered and removal of the whole of the lower lip with a bilateral radical cervical lymph node dissection was not recommended because there was no sign of clinical activity in the lesion of the lip. It was felt better to keep the patient under observation and deal radically with any manifestation which might occur. The patient was referred back to her surgeon.

THE TONGUE
Carcinoma is the usual variety of tumour of the tongue and this disease is now diagnosed in an earlier stage and is becoming less common. This change is due to several factors including the rarity of tertiary syphilis and the decrease in oral leukoplakia. There is now a better standard of oral hygiene and a decrease

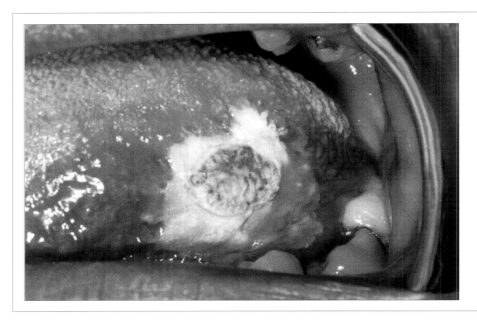

Figure 3 Squamous cell carcinoma in the left lateral border of the tongue surrounded by an area of leukoplakia

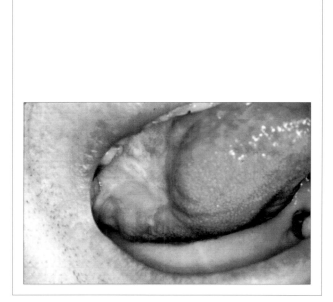

Figure 4 The healed tongue after excision of the carcinoma and area of leukoplakia

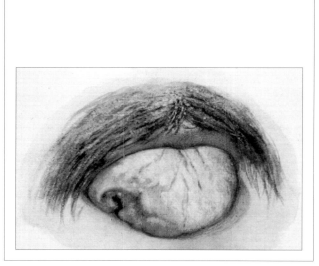

Figure 5 Epithelioma of the tongue associated with syphilitic glossitis (artist's drawing)

in the habit of smoking tobacco in pipes, cigarettes and cigars and of chewing tobacco. There is also a decrease in the harmful habit of the heavy consumption of alcohol associated with smoking tobacco.

Other malignant tumours of the tongue are very rare. An account of these rare tumours in the lips and mouth including the tongue, with references to the literature, was given by Raven[1].

Precancerous lesions
Traumatic lesions
Chronic ulcers in the lateral border of the tongue and in the buccal aspect of the cheek are caused by friction from a jagged tooth or a badly fitting denture; this is the so-called 'dental ulcer'. The edge of the ulcer is hard and indurated and a biopsy is done to eliminate carcinoma, which may supervene if the cause is not removed.

Leukoplakia
This condition affects the mucous membrane of the tongue and other parts of the mouth. The cause may be chronic irritation and some patients, especially with leukoplakia of the anterior part of the dorsum of the tongue, have tertiary syphilis. There may be vitamin A deficiency or no other apparent cause. It is accepted that mouth leukoplakia is precancerous so any obvious cause is treated and patients are kept under observation. A biopsy is done when there is doubtful carcinoma present. This lesion is becoming increasingly uncommon.

Case record A male patient aged 58 years was seen with a superficial squamous cell carcinoma in the left lateral border of the tongue. The carcinoma was surrounded by an area of leukoplakia (Figure 3). Excision of the carcinoma with the leukoplakia was carried out; postoperative radiotherapy to the tongue was given by interstitial radium needles. The patient had no recurrent or metastatic carcinoma 23 years later (Figure 4).

Chronic syphilitic glossitis
In this condition patches of leukoplakia are present on the dorsum of the tongue, which is thickened, fissured and scarred. There is atrophy of the papillae and shiny areas are seen in the mucous membrane (Figure 5). These patients are kept under observation because of the risk of carcinoma which usually is of rapid growth.

Paterson–Kelly syndrome
The association of carcinoma of the mouth with the Paterson–Kelly syndrome is well recognized. There are atrophic and degenerative changes in the mucous membrane of the mouth, including the tongue, and in the pharynx, where malignant changes can supervene. This subject of the Paterson–Kelly syndrome is considered later in a special section.

Carcinoma of the tongue
Carcinoma occurs more often in the tongue than in other sites in the mouth and is usually of the squamous cell type. Males are affected three times more often than females and patients are usually in the sixth decade of life or older. The site of the carcinoma is usually in the lateral border of the middle third of the tongue, followed by the posterior third; the tip, dorsum and under-surface are sometimes affected. In a few patients there is diffuse infiltration of the whole tongue.

Varieties of carcinoma
Malignant ulcer
This is the common variety and has the characteristic features of an epithelioma. In the early stage the edge is raised, hard and indurated; the base is roughened but relatively clean. Initially, there is little invasion of the muscles of the tongue, but later extensive infiltration occurs in the tongue and into the floor of the mouth, alveolus, oropharynx and epiglottis.

Papilliferous tumour
A small swelling develops in the substance of the dorsum or inferior surface of the anterior part of the tongue. This is covered by intact mucous membrane

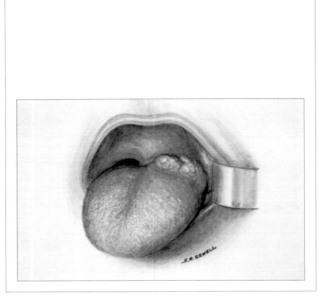

Figure 6 Carcinoma of the tongue invading tonsil and palate (artist's drawing)

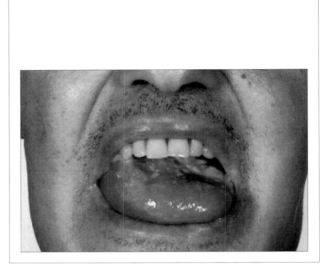

Figure 7 Male with advanced carcinoma of the tongue

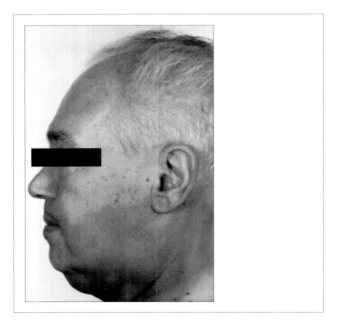

Figure 8 Male with advanced tongue carcinoma and lymph node metastases

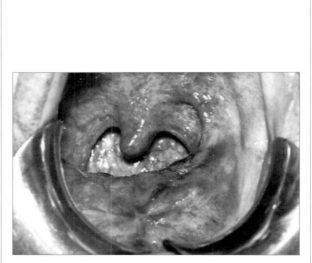

Figure 9 The mouth of a male patient 10 years after total glossectomy for an extensive carcinoma of the tongue. There is no recurrent or metastatic carcinoma. Hypertrophy of the tissues of the floor of the mouth is shown

and gradually enlarges and develops papilliferous processes. Eventually it may become very large; the base is indurated and its surface becomes ulcerated. Sometimes multiple tumours are present separated by apparently normal mucous membrane.

Plaque

There is a flat plaque of carcinoma apparently stuck on the surface of the dorsum of the tongue. It is covered by mucous membrane devoid of papillae and there is some surrounding tissue induration.

Diffuse induration

The whole tongue is diffusely infiltrated by carcinoma causing uniform hardness and perhaps some contraction of the organ. There is considerable fibrosis and tongue movements are impaired.

Carcinoma in a fissure

A carcinoma sometimes develops in the bottom of a chronic fissure in the tongue substance. Whenever a deep fissure is present, the bottom should be inspected for the presence of a carcinoma.

Multiple carcinomas

Occasionally there are multiple carcinomas separated by apparently normal epithelium. As they increase in size coalescence occurs to form a large tumour which almost fills the mouth.

Spread of the carcinoma

Carcinoma of the tongue spreads by direct extension into contiguous tissues in the mouth, oropharynx and epiglottis (Figure 6). Metastases occur in the regional lymph nodes (Figures 7 and 8). Carcinoma of the tip of the tongue affects the submental lymph nodes; of the anterior two-thirds, excluding the tip, metastases occur in the submaxillary and deep cervical lymph nodes; from the posterior third the deep cervical nodes are affected. With a central carcinoma in the tongue, or when a lateral carcinoma extends through the median raphe, metastases may develop in bilateral cervical lymph nodes.

Distant blood-borne metastases may develop in the lung, liver, heart, skeleton and other structures. A second carcinoma is sometimes found in the oesophagus.

Special cases involving carcinoma of the tongue

An account is given here of several special cases of tongue carcinoma which are uncommon.

Total glossectomy

With earlier diagnosis, the development of radiotherapy and present indications for partial glossectomy operations for tongue carcinoma, the operation of total glossectomy is rarely necessary. When extensive carcinoma with diffuse infiltration of the tongue is present, a total glossectomy is carried out if the disease remains operable.

A total glossectomy was performed for a male patient with extensive carcinoma with a good result. Rehabilitation was carried out resulting in very satisfactory speech and mastication and he swallowed his food very well. The patient was alive and well 10 years later and there was no recurrent or metastatic carcinoma (Figure 9).

Carcinoma of the tongue in females

Carcinoma of the tongue is much more frequent in males than in females. Since the disease is uncommon in females the following examples are of interest.

Case record   A female aged 74 years was referred with a carcinoma of the right lateral border of the tongue. A partial glossectomy and a block dissection of the cervical lymph nodes was performed. The patient lived 7 years and 10 months without recurrent or metastatic carcinoma and died aged 82 years of heart failure.

A carcinoma of the posterior third of the tongue may spread by direct extension into the upper part of

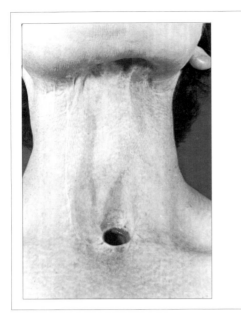

Figure 10 Female aged 49 years following the operation of laryngoglossopharyngectomy for carcinoma of the base of the tongue extending into the epiglottis, uncontrolled by radiotherapy

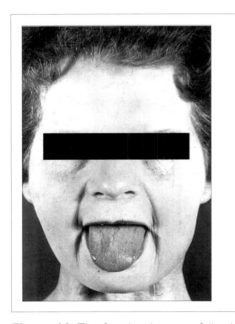

Figure 11 The functional tongue following laryngoglosso-pharyngectomy

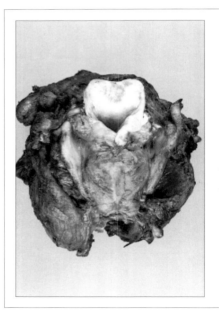

Figure 12 Specimen removed by laryngoglossopharyn-gectomy showing an advanced carcinoma of the base of the tongue extending into the epiglottis

the larynx which creates a difficult treatment problem to solve, especially when radiotherapy fails to control the disease. A patient in this condition was referred for treatment.

Case record A female aged 49 years was referred with an advanced carcinoma of the base of the tongue extending into the epiglottis. She had received a full course of radiotherapy which failed to control the disease and was referred for surgical treatment. The problem was carefully considered and an operation to eradicate the disease and conserve a functional tongue was designed. A laryngoglossopharyngectomy was performed as a one-stage operation. The anterior two-thirds of the tongue and the hypoglossal nerves were conserved; the larynx and part of the hypopharynx were removed and the hypopharynx was reconstructed; a permanent tracheostomy was established (Figures 10–12). Histopathology showed a squamous cell carcinoma. The patient made an excellent recovery with perfect wound healing. The tongue moved normally and was fully functional, and deglutition was normal. The patient was alive and well 17 years and 5 months following surgical treatment and there was no recurrent or metastatic carcinoma.

Betel nut chewing and carcinoma of the tongue

The association of tongue carcinoma and betel nut chewing is well recognized in India but these cases are not seen often in Britain. The case records of two patients who were referred from India for treatment are included here.

Case record A male aged 35 years was referred with a carcinoma of the left lateral border of the tongue, noticed 4 months previously. For many years the patient had chewed betel nut in India. Examination showed an ulcer 0.5 cm in diameter with surrounding induration in the middle third of the left lateral border of the tongue. Histopathology showed a moderately differentiated squamous cell carcinoma.

Treatment was undertaken with a radium needle tongue implant with a tumour dose of 600 R. Seven weeks later wedge excision of the affected area was carried out. Histopathology showed no residual carcinoma. Two weeks later a left radical neck dissection for enlarged left deep cervical and supraclavicular lymph nodes was performed. Histopathology showed no carcinoma in 27 lymph nodes and tuberculosis in the left supraclavicular lymph nodes.

The patient was again referred 24 years later with enlarged mediastinal and retroperitoneal lymph nodes. Histopathology of the mediastinal lymph nodes showed extensive replacement by coalescing epithelioid granuloma with scattered Langhans type giant cells consistent with tuberculosis. A complete course of antituberculosis treatment was given for 9 months and the patient made a good recovery.

The patient continued well until 28 years after his original treatment for tongue carcinoma, when he was referred again for treatment of a swelling he had noticed in the left side of his tongue. Examination showed a round swelling 2 cm in diameter in the left lateral border of the tongue; it was red and firm in consistency. No enlarged cervical or other lymph nodes were noted. A biopsy showed sheets of mainly keratinized pleomorphic malignant squamous cells indicating a squamous cell carcinoma having the appearance of a new primary tumour.

Radiotherapy with a tumour dose of 8180 cGy was followed by a left hemiglossectomy using laser technique. The patient returned to India.

Case record A male aged 34 years from India was referred with a carcinoma of the base of the right side of the tongue. For many years this patient had chewed betel nut, but no tobacco; he had rarely smoked a cigarette and taken alcohol. For 7 years he had had difficulty in opening his mouth and 3 months earlier he had developed pain below the angle of the right mandible which was referred to the floor of the mouth, the right ear and the right upper neck. His surgeon in India found extensive submucous fibrosis of the oral mucous membrane so that the patient was unable to open his mouth to permit examination of his tongue, but a scan showed a suspicious lesion in the base of the right side of the tongue. A general anaesthetic was administered; his mouth could be opened only about 1.5 cm and using a paediatric laryngoscope the surgeon saw a raised indurated slough about 1 cm in diameter in the base of the right side of the tongue extending laterally to the tonsillolingual sulcus and the glossopharyngeal fold. Multiple biopsies showed a moderately differentiated squamous cell carcinoma. The patient was referred for treatment.

Examination showed marked fibrosis of the mucous membrane of both angles of the mouth which prohibited inspection of the tongue, and the finger could not be introduced into the mouth to palpate the carcinoma of the tongue. An enlarged lymph node was present in the right upper neck posterior to the angle of the mandible.

A review of the histopathology showed small biopsies invaded by a squamous cell carcinoma forming some keratin, but with other foci showing poor differentiation. Some of the superficial squamous mucosa showed severe dysplasia. The depth of invasion could not be assessed in these small fragments and no muscle was included, but the sections were consistent with being from the tongue.

Treatment options were discussed between the surgeon and radiotherapist and a decision was made to treat this tongue carcinoma with external beam radiotherapy (photons) to include the oropharynx, sparing the incisor teeth, but including the anterior cervical, posterior cervical and the supraclavicular lymph nodes in both sides of the neck. This treatment was completed with a dosage of 6000 cGy. Adequate nourishment throughout the patient's treatment was ensured.

The enlarged upper deep right cervical lymph node was used as an external marker for changes in the primary tongue carcinoma, which could not be observed or palpated because the patient was unable to open his mouth sufficiently for this examination. This enlarged lymph node regressed during treatment and became very small and soft in consistency. It was considered that this reflected regression in the primary carcinoma also.

The patient returned to India to continue under careful supervision.

THE FLOOR OF THE MOUTH

Carcinoma is the commonest tumour to occur in the floor of the mouth although other rare tumours have been described. These include the mixed salivary gland tumour and the plasma cell tumours.

Carcinoma

Carcinoma, usually squamous cell in type, occurs primarily in the floor of the mouth or spreads there by direct extension from a carcinoma in the tongue.

Special reference is made to the association of smoking a clay pipe with the development of carcinoma in the floor of the mouth at the site of impingement of the stem of the pipe causing chronic irritation. This habit has practically disappeared so the following illustration is of historic interest.

Case record A male patient, after smoking a clay pipe for many years, developed a squamous cell carcinoma in the floor of the mouth at the site where the stem of the pipe impinged. The carcinoma was extensive and spread to the alveolus and the left mandible. Treatment was by wide excision of the carcinoma and the surrounding tissues in the floor of the mouth together with the horizontal ramus of the left mandible. The wound healed well and the patient was free of recurrent and metastatic carcinoma 2 years and 2 months later (Figures 13–16).

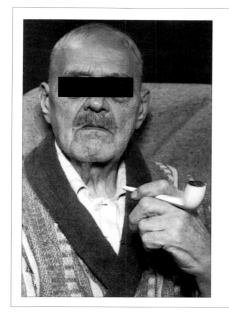

Figure 13 Male who smoked a clay pipe for many years

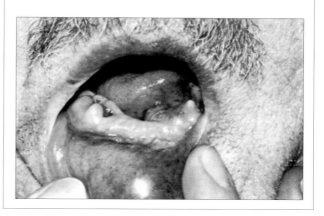

Figure 14 Extensive squamous carcinoma in the floor of the mouth where the pipe stem impinged. The carcinoma spread to the left alveolus and mandible

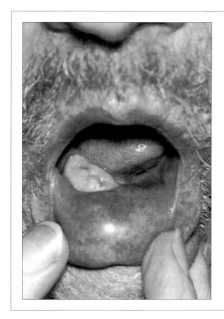

Figure 15 The healed floor of the mouth following wide excision of the carcinoma and horizontal ramus of the left mandible

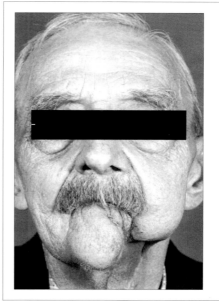

Figure 16 Appearance following excision; no recurrent or metastatic carcinoma 2 years and 2 months later

Varieties of carcinoma

Malignant ulcer

This is the usual variety which occurs in the region of the frenum linguae or at the orifice of Wharton's duct. The initial ulcer shows no sign of healing, gradually increases in size and has all the characteristic features of a carcinomatous ulcer.

Papilliferous tumour

This commences as a nodule and is covered by mucous membrane. It gradually increases in size, papilliferous processes are formed, the base is indurated and superficial ulceration occurs.

Diffuse carcinoma

The whole of the floor of the mouth is diffusely infiltrated by the carcinoma causing the tissues to be hard and unyielding to the touch. There is little or no ulceration.

Spread of the carcinoma

Carcinoma of the floor of the mouth spreads by direct extension in all directions to the under-surface of the tongue, alveolus, and mandible, fauces and tonsil and the lower lip. Metastases occur in the submental and submaxillary lymph nodes, unilaterally or bilaterally according to the position of the primary tumour in the floor of the mouth. Later, metastases develop in the deep cervical lymph nodes and rarely in the pre-auricular lymph nodes.

Treatment

Carcinoma in the floor of the mouth which does not involve the mandible or regional lymph nodes is usually treated with radiotherapy, but if the tumour is not controlled and lymph node metastases are present, surgical treatment is necessary.

The result achieved by combined radiation and surgical treatment is shown in the following case report.

Case record A female aged 40 years was referred with an extensive carcinoma in the floor of the mouth reaching from the left side across the midline for about 1 cm. It measured 5 × 2.5 cm anteroposteriorly and involved the under-surface of the tongue and the mucous membrane of the inner side of the mandible (Figure 17). Movements of the tongue were limited and there was induration in the left submandibular region extending into the right side. There was an enlarged hard lymph node 1 cm in diameter in the left submandibular region and a small hard lymph node in the left upper deep cervical group. A radiogram of the left mandible showed no bone erosion.

The patient was treated with pre-operative radiotherapy; a tumour dose of 600 R was given. There was some tumour regression but considerable induration remained. A monoblock excision of the floor of the mouth and inferior aspect of the tongue was then performed combined with a left radical suprahyoid lymph node dissection and a modified upper right cervical lymph node dissection (Figure 18). Subsequently the floor of the mouth was reconstructed in stages using the tongue for the inner aspect. Outer skin cover was obtained by acromiopectoral tubed pedicle skin grafts. Perfect healing occurred (Figure 19). On histopathology, the oral tissues showed a well-differentiated squamous cell carcinoma growing in an abundant densely collagenized fibroblastic stroma, deep to the surface epithelium. The planes of surgical excision were clear by wide margins. There were no metastases in the lymph nodes.

The patient was well and there was no recurrent or metastatic carcinoma 21 years later. She could eat satisfactorily, and could speak well even on the telephone.

THE ALVEOLUS

Carcinoma

Carcinoma is the usual tumour that occurs in the

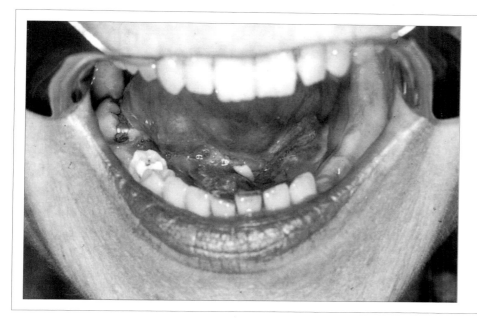

Figure 17 Female with an extensive squamous cell carcinoma in the floor of the mouth involving the under-surface of the tongue and the mucous membrane on the inner side of the mandible

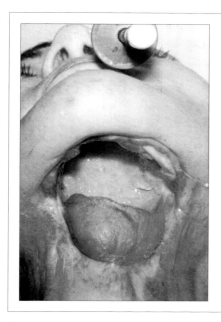

Figure 18 After excision of the floor of the mouth. The illustration shows the soft tissue defect in the floor of the mouth, including the submandibular skin, allowing the tongue to prolapse into the neck

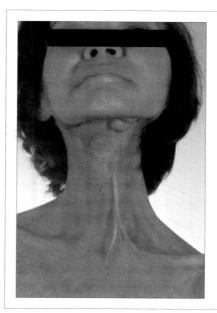

Figure 19 After the reconstruction of the floor of the mouth and the submandibular defect, showing perfect healing 8 months later

alveolus and this may be primary in this situation, or a carcinoma in a neighbouring structure such as the floor of the mouth, tongue, lip, oropharynx or the antrum of Highmore.

The tumour commences as a small ulcer or nodule in the mucous membrane of the gum. The presence of a loose tooth may call the attention of the patient to the carcinoma, and bleeding may occur.

Spread of the disease

As the carcinoma increases in size, local proliferation occurs and contiguous tissues are invaded including the underlying bone of the maxilla or mandible and the antrum of Highmore.

Metastases occur in the regional lymph nodes in the submental, submaxillary and deep cervical groups.

Treatment

For a primary carcinoma confined to the mucous membrane of the alveolus, a course of radiotherapy is given. If the tumour proves radioresistant, wide excision is performed.

When the carcinoma is invading the underlying bone, a radical surgical excision is performed according to the extent of the disease. A localized tumour is removed with a wedge resection of the underlying alveolar process of the jaw. For an extensive carcinoma of the lower alveolus a resection of the horizontal ramus or hemimandibulectomy is required performed in continuity with a block dissection of the regional lymph nodes as a monoblock operation. When the maxilla is affected by an extensive carcinoma, for example when the antrum of Highmore is invaded, a resection of the maxilla is required. The following case record concerns a patient who was referred for treatment of an extensive carcinoma of the alveolus.

Case record   A female aged 47 years was referred with a carcinoma involving the left lower alveolus.

Examination showed a proliferative variety of carcinoma 5 × 2 cm affecting the left lower alveolus, fixed to the mandible but not invading the floor of the mouth. The submental, submaxillary and upper deep cervical lymph nodes were enlarged, hard and a little fixed. A radiograph of the left mandible showed considerable absorption of the alveolar edge of the molar region and some rarefaction posterior to this near the base of the coronoid process.

A monoblock excision was performed, including a left radical neck dissection, right submental lymph node excision, resection of the left mandible from the angle to the symphysis menti, and excision of the mucosa of the left floor of the mouth. The left mandible was reconstructed with a polythene prosthesis but this was extruded 3 years later (Figures 20–22).

Histopathology showed an active keratinizing squamous cell carcinoma of the alveolus. Metastases were present in the submental and two upper cervical lymph nodes.

The patient was well 30 years later and there was no recurrent or metastatic carcinoma.

Malignant melanoma

Malignant melanoma of the alveolus is an extremely rare tumour and has a grave prognosis.

Case record   A patient was referred with a malignant melanoma which occurred in a deep tooth socket of the left lower jaw in a male aged 27 years. The tooth had been removed and the socket appeared to have healed but there was a bluish-black discoloration in the centre of the socket and a swelling posteriorly in the alveolar margin, hard in consistency and covered by mucous membrane. The horizontal ramus of the left mandible was excised and a radical dissection of the left cervical lymph nodes and dissection of the upper right cervical lymph nodes was performed. Histopathology of the tumour of the left alveolus

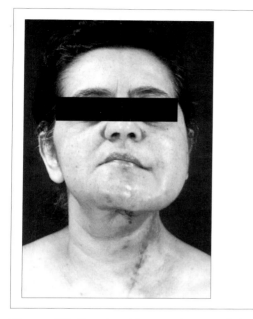

Figure 20 Female with a carcinoma of the left alveolus invading the left mandible with metastases in the regional lymph nodes after left mandibulectomy, left radical neck dissection and the insertion of a polythene prosthesis to replace the left mandible

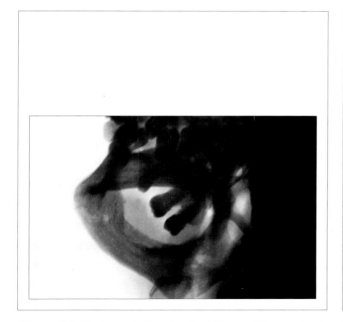

Figure 21 Radiograph showing the left mandible prosthesis

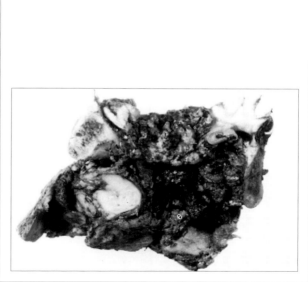

Figure 22 Specimen showing the squamous cell carcinoma of the left alveolus infiltrating the left mandible and metastases in the left submental and upper deep cervical lymph nodes

showed the submucosa to be occupied by a highly cellular malignant melanoma. Pigment was prominent in places. In one area there was some functional activity indicating a local origin.

During the subsequent 1 year and 5 months melanoma recurred in the mouth and right sub-mandibular region.

Cylindroma

A cylindroma (adenoid cystic carcinoma) sometimes occurs in the buccal aspect of the cheek and forms metastases in the regional cervical lymph nodes and may disseminate more widely. This carries a serious prognosis and requires radical excision.

Case record A female aged 67 years had for about 1 year noticed a swelling in the posterior aspect of the left lower alveolus which at first was intermittent and later fixed. Examination showed a proliferative tumour of the left lower alveolus behind the second molar tooth 2 cm in diameter, fixed to the mandible and filling the retromolar sulcus surrounding the third molar tooth (Figure 23). The left submental and submaxillary lymph nodes were enlarged. A biopsy showed the structure of a cylindroma.

The patient underwent preoperative radiotherapy with a tumour dose of 5350 R. An excision of the alveolus tumour through a left submandibular incision was then performed. The tumour was localized to the mucosa and had not invaded bone, and was excised with a margin of surrounding mucosa. The left second and third molar teeth were extracted. Bone chips were removed from the underlying bone for histopathology. Frozen section histology of lymph nodes showed no carcinoma.

Sections through the centre and lateral edges of the main tumour showed infiltration of the tissue beneath and around the area of ulceration by cylindroma (adenoid cystic carcinoma) of mucous gland origin. The tumour tissue showed marked irradiation

changes and was present as small cystic structures in a fibrocellular stroma. The lateral lines of excision were free of tumour but on the deep surface where the tissue was dissected from bone, tumour extended to the edge of the tissue received for examination. The multiple fragments of bone were tumour-free. Lymph nodes showed no metastases.

There was no recurrent or metastatic carcinoma $2\frac{1}{2}$ months later (Figure 24).

THE CHEEK

Carcinoma of the buccal aspect of the cheek

Carcinoma arising in the mucous membrane of the buccal aspect of the cheek is a serious disease for it causes considerable deformity of the face, especially when the angle of the mouth is affected, and poses difficult treatment problems.

The tumour is usually a squamous cell carcinoma and spreads by direct extension in the soft tissues of the cheek. Metastases also occur in the regional lymph nodes in the neck. Regarding the treatment, radiotherapy is carefully considered and is usually given as the primary treatment. When radiotherapy fails to control the carcinoma, surgical treatment is required. Recurrent carcinoma here creates a serious situation where regional perfusion of the tumour with chemotherapy has been used with a remarkable result.

Case record A female aged 53 years was referred with a carcinoma of the buccal aspect of the left cheek which was uncontrolled by radiotherapy (tumour dose 5000 R) in another country. Histopathology showed a well differentiated squamous cell carcinoma. The patient gave the history that over a 2-year period she had continuously injured her left cheek with her upper denture when eating. A small superficial ulcer had appeared which gradually increased in size. Two months earlier this ulcer had been shown

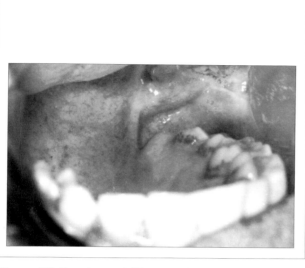

Figure 23 Female aged 67 years with a cylindroma of the left lower alveolus behind the second molar tooth

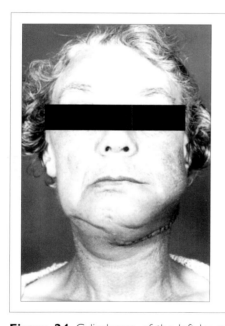

Figure 24 Cylindroma of the left lower alveolus excised through a left mandibular incision; the healed wound

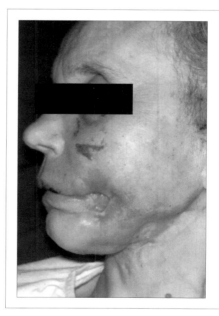

Figure 25 Female aged 53 years with a recurrent squamous cell carcinoma of the left cheek following radiotherapy and surgical treatment. The carcinoma involved the whole thickness of the cheek

by histology to be a squamous cell highly differentiated carcinoma; in some areas keratinized pearls were present with only a few mitoses. The tumour had been treated with radiotherapy but had not been controlled and it had increased in size.

Examination showed a carcinoma in the buccal aspect of the left cheek 6 × 5 cm with a central necrotic slough; it extended to the alveolus but the bone seemed unaffected. The overlying facial skin was reddened over an area of 2.5 cm where it was attached to the tumour on the left angle of the mouth. The left submental lymph node was firm in consistency.

The carcinoma of the buccal aspect of the left cheek was excised through a submandibular approach, removing an area of skin on the left angle of the mouth, combined with a left suprahyoid lymph node dissection. The defect in the cheek mucous membrane was repaired with a flap of mucous membrane raised from the mouth floor and the facial skin wound was sutured. The patient made a good recovery and the wounds healed well (Figure 25). Histopathology showed a well differentiated squamous cell carcinoma extending through the cheek muscle to within 1 mm of the surface of the specimen. An upper deep cervical lymph node contained a metastasis.

A course of postoperative radiotherapy was given to the affected area in a dose of 3000 R.

Six months later the patient returned with a large recurrent carcinoma involving the whole thickness of the left cheek over an extensive area. This condition caused a very difficult treatment problem following radiotherapy and surgery.

A decision was made to carry out an intra-arterial tumour perfusion after introducing the catheter through the superficial temporal artery into the external carotid artery at the correct site for the perfusion,

determined by injecting dye to outline the soft tissues of the left side of the face. A total dose of 350 mg methotrexate and 7.5 mg nitrogen mustard was perfused into the tumour over a period of 2 weeks. There was an immediate and remarkable regression of the tumour, which seemed to melt away completely leaving a soft tissue defect at the left angle of the mouth (Figure 26). This defect was reconstructed surgically 3 months later and the wound healed well (Figure 27).

The patient was well and there was no recurrent or metastatic carcinoma 16 years later.

THE PALATE

Carcinoma

Carcinoma is the usual tumour that occurs in the palate but it is not common. A primary carcinoma may develop in either the hard or soft palate, but the palate is also affected secondarily by a carcinoma in an adjacent structure. Thus, a primary carcinoma of the alveolus, oropharynx (tonsil or faucial pillars) or nasopharynx spreads by direct extension into the soft palate. A carcinoma in the antrum of Highmore spreads downwards to affect both the hard and soft palate.

A primary carcinoma of the palate commences as an ulcer or lump which gradually enlarges; bleeding may occur and teeth in the upper jaw become loose.

A carcinomatous ulcer with the usual characteristics is the most common variety; sometimes a papilliferous tumour occurs which gradually enlarges and later becomes ulcerated; the base is indurated.

Spread of the disease

This occurs by direct extension and in the hard palate the underlying bone is infiltrated. Metastases may develop in the regional lymph nodes.

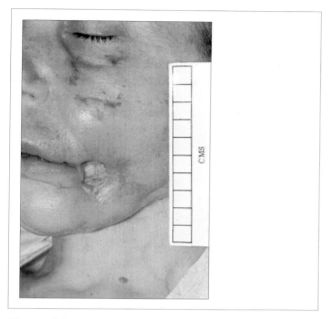

Figure 26 The marked regression following regional perfusion chemotherapy

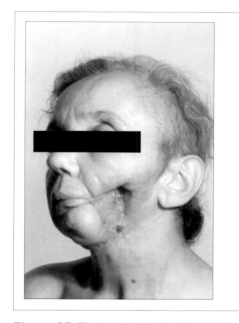

Figure 27 The healed cheek after reconstruction surgery

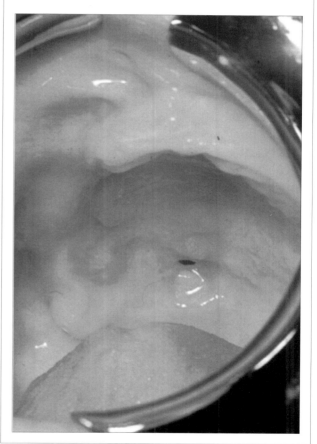

Figure 28 Patient with a cylindroma in the right side of the palate showing the raised tumour covered by mucous membrane

Treatment

Carcinoma of the soft palate is treated with radio-therapy, but if the tumour proves radioresistant or recurs, radical excision of the soft palate is carried out. A small carcinoma (less than 2.5 cm in diameter) of the hard palate is given preoperative radiotherapy. When complete regression of the tumour does not occur, wide surgical excision including the underlying bone involvement, so a partial resection of the maxilla including the whole tumour area is performed.

Cylindroma

A cylindroma is not uncommon in the palate. An example is shown in Figure 28.

REFERENCE

1. Raven, R. W. (1958). *Malignant tumours of the lips and mouth*. In *Cancer*, Vol. 4, ch. 2. (London: Butterworth & Co. Ltd.)

2

Tumours of the jaws

Tumours of the jaws, apart from involvement by tumours in the mouth, nose and accessory air sinuses including the antrum of Highmore, are rare. It should be noted that dental structures in the jaws may give rise to benign or malignant tumours.

Malignant tumours that arise in the jaws themselves are similar to other bone tumours such as myeloma, osteogenic sarcomas and other varieties of sarcoma, and illustrations of these tumours are given in Chapter 17.

Illustrations of involvement of the jaws by malignant tumours in different parts of the mouth are given in the appropriate sections. An additional illustration is shown in Figures 1 and 2 of a highly cellular carcinoma which developed in the buccal aspect of the left cheek in a very short period of several weeks and invaded the right mandible by direct extension.

Primary tumours with a propensity to metastasize to bones in general can also form metastases in the jaws, but such metastases are uncommon.

EMBRYONAL SARCOMA OF THE MANDIBLE

This tumour is rare in the mandible. The following case history is a remarkable example in that the size of the tumour and the severe deformity it caused in the child's face were very impressive, together with the long survival period following treatment without recurrent or metastatic disease.

Case record A male child aged $3\frac{1}{2}$ years was referred from another country. Two years previously he had banged the right side of his face on the corner of a table which had caused bruising, and nine months previously he had fallen from a chair and had banged the same place, which had become swollen. The swelling had developed to the size of an egg. A biopsy had been done which had revealed an embryonal sarcoma. A course of radiotherapy had been given to the tumour which had then measured 5 × 7 × 3 cm; the tumour dose was 4600 R. There had been some initial tumour regression and then it had continued to enlarge.

Examination showed a well-developed healthy boy aged $3\frac{1}{2}$ years. A large tumour projected from the right side of his face causing a severe deformity (Figure 3). It extended from the temporal fossa to the angle of the mandible and from the pinna to the side of his nose; the tumour measured 13.8 × 11.2 cm. The tumour was lobulated, semifluctant and not tender. On palpation through the mouth the tumour was noted to be lateral to the maxilla and the palate felt normal. The skin of the face was normal. No enlarged lymph nodes were found in the neck. Histopathology showed the tumour to be an embryonal

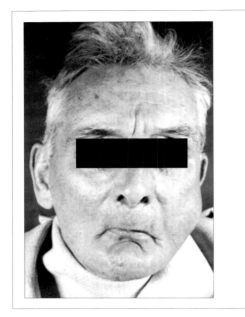

Figure 1 Male aged 71 years showing deformity of the left side of the face caused by a highly cellular carcinoma of the buccal aspect of the cheek which invaded the left mandible

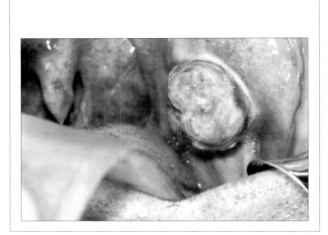

Figure 2 The tumour in the same patient

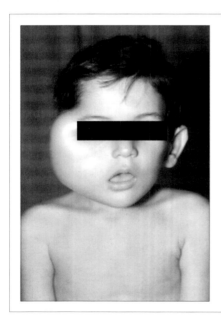

Figure 3 Male child aged 3½ years with a large embryonal sarcoma projecting from the right face

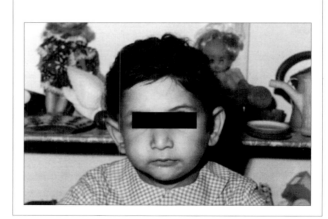

Figure 4 The results achieved 1½ years after combined radiotherapy and chemotherapy. Chemotherapy was continued with actinomycin D, vincristine and cyclophosphamide. At the age of 5½ years there was no evidence of the primary tumour, or metastases

sarcoma. Cross-striations were not demonstrated but it was considered that the tumour was liable to behave as an embryonal rhabdomyosarcoma.

Tomograms of the skull showed the right petrous bone and mastoid process to be normal. Almost the whole of the ascending ramus of the mandible including the condyle on the right side had been destroyed by the tumour. The lateral wall of the right antrum and the posterior part of the alveolar portion of the right maxilla had also been destroyed. There was evidence of destruction of the lateral wall of the right orbit and of the inferior wall of the orbit and malar bone. Chest X-ray showed no evidence of metastases or other abnormality.

The patient was treated with a course of radiotherapy with a total maximum tumour dose of 4732 R. This was followed by chemotherapy: thiotepa 15 mg injected into the tumour and vincristine 1.0 mg, adriamycin 10 mg, methotrexate 5 mg and bleomycin 5 mg given intramuscularly; two doses were administered. There was regression of the tumour both externally and in the mouth. The patient then returned to his country to continue chemotherapy with methotrexate.

On returning to Britain for follow-up he was given further chemotherapy and 7 months after his first treatment his face was almost normal. Maintenance chemotherapy with cyclophosphamide was arranged when he returned home. On his periodic visits to Britain he was given a course of actinomycin and vincristine. Chemotherapy ceased 3 years and 4 months after the first treatment (Figure 4). The patient was well at age 19 years, 16 years after treatment, and there was no recurrent or metastatic embryonal sarcoma.

CARCINOMA OF THE JAW

A squamous cell carcinoma which arises in the substance of the jaw causes it to expand and the teeth become loose. The tumour spreads by direct extension through the bone and ulcerates into the mouth or through the skin of the face causing severe deformity. Metastases may develop in the cervical lymph nodes and through the bloodstream into viscera such as the lungs.

Case record A male aged 44 years was referred with an advanced squamous cell carcinoma of the right maxilla. This extensive tumour had progressed externally to cause a severe facial deformity with ulceration of the skin, and had spread into the right orbital tissues including the lower eyelid and the side of the nose (Figure 5). The carcinoma had been treated by radiotherapy in another country. There was no evidence of metastases. The treatment was carefully considered and because further radiotherapy was not possible a radical surgical excision including the right maxilla, eye with the lower eyelid and part of the orbit was performed (Figure 6). Following the operation the patient was fitted with a good facial prosthesis (Figure 7).

Subsequently the patient developed recurrent disease in the region of the right mandible and metastases in the right submandibular lymph nodes and right frontal bone with involvement of the frontal sinus, 8 months after the operation. He was treated with radiotherapy.

The patient continued to be ambulant and wore his prosthesis which was comfortable and helpful. He died 1 year and 2 months after his initial operation.

Histopathology of the radical excision specimen of the advanced squamous cell carcinoma of the right maxilla showed the tumour to be a well differentiated squamous cell carcinoma, extensively invading the tissues of the cheek. It was present in the masseter muscle at the level of the second lower molar tooth, the temporal muscle, the pterygoid muscle, the posterior margin of the orbit and orbital tissues, and the lower eyelid.

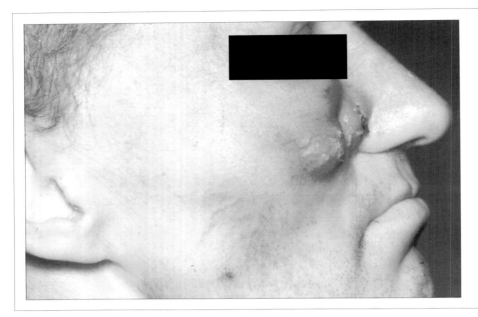

Figure 5 Male aged 44 years with an extensive squamous cell carcinoma causing severe facial deformity with skin ulceration, and involving the right orbital tissues including the lower eyelid and side of the nose

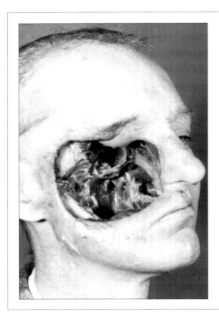

Figure 6 The same patient following radical surgical excision including the right maxilla, eye with the lower eyelid and part of the orbit

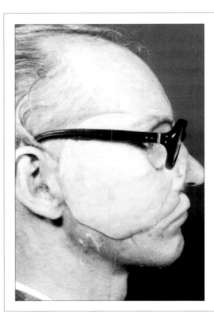

Figure 7 The patient wearing his facial prosthesis

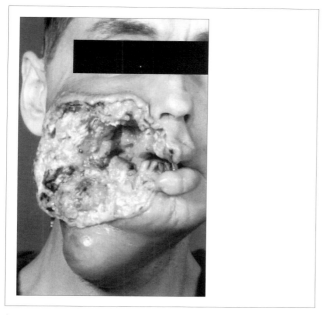

Figure 8 Male patient with an advanced carcinoma of both jaws destroying the right cheek, causing severe deformity of the face and extending into the lymph nodes and tissues in the right submaxillary region

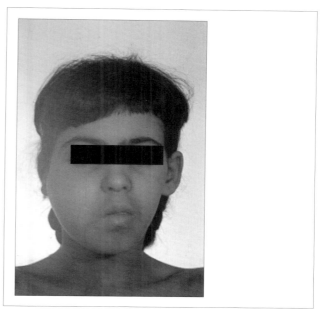

Figure 9 Male patient with a rhabdomyosarcoma of the right side of his face

Case record A patient was referred with a massive carcinoma involving both the upper and lower right jaws; it had extended widely to destroy the tissues of the right cheek, angle of the mouth and part of the upper and lower lips. The carcinoma had spread into the lymph nodes and other tissues of the right submaxillary region which were covered by very thin skin about to ulcerate (Figure 8). This extensive carcinoma was inoperable.

It is fortunate that these patients are seen today before such widespread carcinoma develops.

RHABDOMYOSARCOMA OF THE MAXILLA

Rhabdomyosarcoma is a rare tumour of the maxilla. Figure 9 shows a patient referred from another country with this type of lesion. The tumour had caused a marked degree of swelling and deformity of the right side of his face.

3

Tumours of the salivary glands

Tumours of the salivary glands are usually classified according to their histological characteristics rather than whether they are benign or malignant. Some of these tumours are of doubtful or low malignancy; others infiltrate contiguous tissues and structures continuously without giving rise to metastases, whilst there are tumours which have high malignant potential. There are adenomas and adenolymphomas of the salivary glands which are benign. The general term 'salivary glands' includes not only the parotid, submaxillary and sublingual glands, but also small salivary glands that occur in the mucous membrane of the palate, lips, cheeks and tongue. Several tumours originating in this salivary gland tissue are described in other sections of this book. In this section tumours of the parotid and submaxillary salivary glands will be illustrated. Regarding their site frequency, tumours of the parotid salivary gland are more frequent than those of the submaxillary salivary gland; the former gland is much larger than the latter and it is situated in a dangerous site when malignant tissue invasion occurs.

The following varieties of salivary gland tumours can be distinguished according to their histopathology.

MIXED TUMOURS

These tumours are more frequent in the parotid than in the submaxillary salivary gland. They gradually increase in size and infiltrate local tissues. Unless they are carefully and completely excised, they rapidly recur and infiltrate but they do not usually metastasize. These tumours should be excised with a reasonable margin of parotid glandular tissue as soon as they are diagnosed.

The histology is somewhat complex with epithelial components forming alveoli, cell strands or cell masses, and mesoblastic tissue forming cartilage, hyaline or myxoid connective tissue, or mucous tissue. Recurrent tumours are more cellular and malignant. In primary mixed salivary gland tumours it is very difficult to differentiate those which are benign from those which have undergone malignant change.

CYLINDROMA

A cylindroma must be regarded as potentially malignant. Histologically the tumour consists of broad columns of epithelial cells which are surrounded by hyaline sheaths. There are two types of cells in these columns, namely cubical or columnar cells lining the small tubules, and smaller myo-epithelial cells. Accumulations of hyaline material are found amongst the cell columns in addition to forming the sheath around them; sometimes mucoid material is present instead of the hyaline matrix. In the tumours which are obviously malignant, the cells are larger and hyperchromatic showing numerous mitoses, and there may be necrosis at the centre of the cell masses.

Widespread local infiltration by the tumour may occur into soft tissues and bone including the skull. The facial nerve becomes paralysed. Metastases in lymph nodes are uncommon.

MUCO-EPIDERMOID TUMOUR

This variety of salivary gland tumour occurs in the small salivary glands in addition to the parotid and submaxillary glands. On histological examination there are cystic spaces which are lined by goblet cells and there are large areas of epidermoid epithelium. In well differentiated tumours there are large mucoid cysts and mucus extravasations may occur into the tissues.

The cut surface of the tumour may reveal cystic spaces full of mucus. The more malignant variety tends to be larger with fewer mucous cysts and infiltrates extensively; these tumours can quite frequently cause metastases in the regional lymph nodes and also in distant viscera.

OTHER CARCINOMAS

These tumours are uncommon. Rarely a squamous cell carcinoma occurs, composed of islands of epidermoid cells in a fibrous stroma; these are very malignant. Another variety is the muco-epidermoid tumour which is composed of glandular spaces lined by goblet cells. This tumour, a mucoid adenocarcinoma, forms lymph node and blood-borne metastases.

CONNECTIVE TISSUE TUMOURS

Benign connective tissue tumours such as haemangioma, lipoma and neurilemmoma are very rare in the parotid and submaxillary salivary glands. Sarcomas of any variety are also extremely rare.

Illustrations

Case record A female aged 27 years was referred from another country with a swelling in the left parotid region which had increased in size for about 3 years. A biopsy had been performed and exploration had shown a hard nodular tumour, with small cystic areas, in the deeper part of the left parotid salivary gland; it was infiltrating the superficial aspect of the underlying mandible. Histopathology showed a muco-epidermoid tumour of the parotid salivary gland.

On examination a hard fixed tumour of the left parotid salivary gland 5 cm in diameter, not attached to skin but firmly attached to the deep structures was found. There was impairment of facial nerve function. Cervical lymph nodes were not enlarged.

The patient was given a course of pre-operative radiotherapy with a tumour dose of about 4500 R. There was no marked tumour regression (Figure 1) and a decision was made to perform a left total parotidectomy after careful consideration; it was anticipated that the left facial nerve would be sacrificed and this was explained to the patient.

Access to the parotid gland was through the previous scar and an extensive fixed tumour with areas of cystic and mucoid degeneration was found, firmly fixed to the ascending ramus of the left mandible. The main left facial nerve was identified. The mandibular and cervical branches were involved in the tumour, and they were divided. The motor branches to the left eye region were identified and conserved although they were stretched. The tumour was carefully dissected out, the affected area of the ascending ramus of the mandible was removed and the deep tumour extension down to the lateral wall of the oropharynx was excised. There was another deep extension into the pterygoid region which was also removed. The styloid process was dissected clean from the tumour.

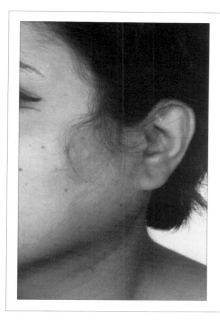

Figure 1 Female aged 27 years with a muco-epidermoid carcinoma of the left parotid salivary gland after exploration and pre-operative radiotherapy; her condition before radical parotidectomy and postoperative radiotherapy is illustrated

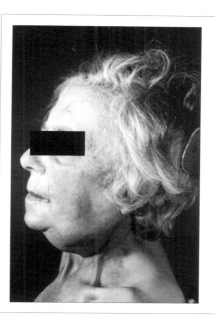

Figure 2 Female aged 75 years with a mixed tumour of the left parotid salivary gland which had been present since she was aged 15 years and had become malignant and inoperable. The tumour extended from the left submaxillary region to the left mastoid process and the pre-auricular region. It was tethered to the mandible

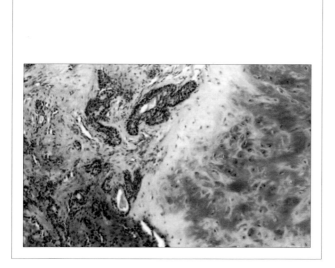

Figure 3 Histopathology of the mixed tumour of the parotid salivary gland in the same patient. In many areas there are groups of polygonal tumour cells which are hyperchromatic and fairly numerous

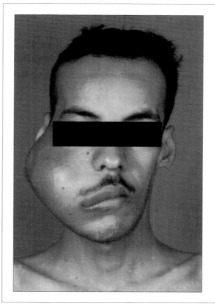

Figure 4 Male with a massive fibrosarcoma of the right parotid salivary gland expanding the right cheek, extending throughout the pre-auricular region and posteriorly below the pinna to the mastoid region. The overlying skin is stretched and red in colour. The tumour has invaded the right mandible

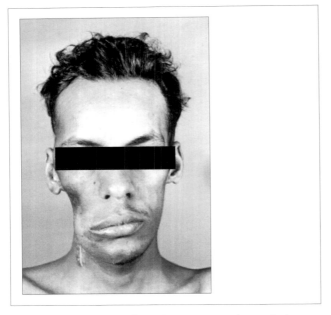

Figure 5 The patient following pre-operative radiotherapy and total parotidectomy combined with a hemimandibulectomy

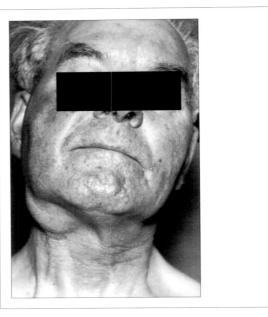

Figure 6 Male aged 66 years with a cylindroma of the right submaxillary salivary gland treated by surgical excision

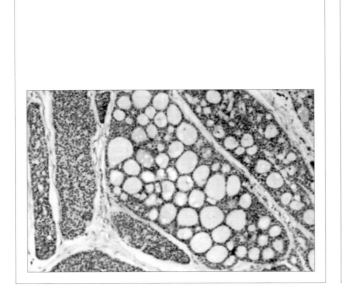

Figure 7 Histopathology of the cylindroma showing the broad columns of epithelial cells which are surrounded by hyaline sheaths

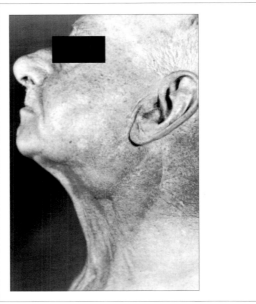

Figure 8 Male with a large fixed infiltrating carcinoma of the left submaxillary salivary gland

The pathology specimen consisted of a block including the parotid salivary gland replaced by firm tumour tissue with soft mucoid areas. The tumour measured 4.5 × 2.8 × 3 cm and reached the cranial and anterior surfaces of the block. Two lymph nodes were present in the caudal end of the specimen. The posterior surface of the excision which included fat with lymph nodes and fragments of muscle was well away from the infiltrating tumour.

Histopathology revealed the tumour to be a muco-epidermoid carcinoma reaching the anterior, cranial and medial lines of resection in the main specimen, but well away from the posterior end. None of the lymph nodes dissected contained metastases. Tumour, surrounded by marked fibrosis, was present within cancellous bone of the ramus of the mandible. Tumour was present in the pterygoid extension and in the tissue from above the styloid process.

Postoperative radiotherapy was given to increase the total dose to 6500 R. The patient subsequently had plastic surgery for the left facial paralysis; she developed a little movement in the left side of her face and could close the left upper eyelid about 75%. She was well with no recurrent or metastatic disease 7 years and 8 months later.

Case record   A female aged 75 years had had a lump in the left side of her face since the age of 15 years. Recently this had become larger and seemed to be extending into the lower jaw and causing increasing pain.

On examination the patient was frail and old with active Parkinson's disease. In the left submaxillary region and extending to the left mastoid process there was a tumour 7 × 5 cm, tethered to the horizontal ramus of the left mandible and extending up into the pre-auricular region where there was marked induration. The overlying skin was normal and both facial nerves were normal (Figure 2).

A biopsy had been performed in another hospital. Histopathology showed the appearance of a mixed salivary gland tumour. In many areas there were groups of polygonal tumour cells which were hyperchromatic and fairly numerous (Figure 3).

A course of radiotherapy with a total dose of 4000 R was given. This resulted in tumour regression to 6 × 4 cm with complete resolution of the induration over the left mandible. No enlarged lymph nodes were found in the neck. After 6 months the patient's general condition was deteriorating. This tumour which had been present for 60 years had become malignant and inoperable.

Case record   Fibrosarcoma is a very rare tumour in the salivary glands. Figures 4 and 5 show a male patient who was referred from another country with this tumour. The patient received a course of radiotherapy and a total parotidectomy combined with a hemimandibulectomy was performed.

Case record   A male aged 66 years had a swelling in the right submaxillary region for 18 months which was gradually increasing in size and was painful at times. Examination showed a hard, lobulated tumour in the right submaxillary region which was mobile and not attached to the skin (Figure 6). No enlarged cervical lymph nodes were noted. The tumour of the right submaxillary salivary gland was excised. On histopathology, the structure was that of a cylindroma of the submaxillary salivary gland (Figure 7).

Figure 8 shows a patient with a large fixed infiltrating carcinoma of the left submaxillary salivary gland.

4

Tumours of the pharynx

The pharynx is affected by both benign and malignant tumours which differ considerably in their frequency, pathology and response to treatment. Anatomically the pharynx is in a relatively inaccessible position, being a musculomembranous tube extending from the base of the skull to the lower border of the cricoid cartilage opposite the intervertebral disc between the 5th and 6th cervical vertebrae. Consequently, there are difficulties in the diagnosis, treatment and subsequent observation of the tumors situated there. The tumour is sometimes extensive when diagnosed and the prognosis following treatment is often poor.

The pharynx is divided into three parts: the nasopharynx (epipharynx) is situated above the soft palate; the oropharynx (mesopharynx) is situated between the soft palate and the hyoid bone; and the hypopharynx. Tumours which occur in each division will be described.

TUMOURS OF THE NASOPHARYNX

Benign tumour
Fibroma
This tumour is uncommon in the nasopharynx; the author has seen it in three patients aged 11, 14 and 15 years. The tumour is usually found in young males, causing nasal obstruction and epistaxis. Other symptoms include supra-orbital headache, deafness and nasal swelling. Nasopharyngeal endoscopy reveals the tumour.

Appearance   The tumour is fleshy and its colour varies from white to red. Large blood vessels are present so that serious haemorrhage may be caused by trauma, including biopsy.

Treatment   A course of radiotherapy is given which reduces the vascularity of the tumour; excision is usually necessary after radiotherapy. Small tumours are removed through the anterior nares, or through the mouth behind the soft palate. Haemorrhage, however slight, must be controlled and postoperative observation is essential to detect bleeding into the bronchial tree or oedema of the glottis.

For a large fibroma, the transpalatal operation is necessary for excision as described by C. P. Wilson[1].

Prognosis   The tumour does not metastasize, but may recur locally.

Malignant tumours
Carcinoma
A squamous cell carcinoma is the commonest malignant tumour in the nasopharynx. There are two varieties: a malignant ulcer and a papilliferous, fleshy, friable tumour projecting into the cavity of the nasopharynx. The surface becomes ulcerated when the

tumour is large. Metastases occur in the retropharyngeal and cervical lymph nodes and in the lungs and liver. Direct extension of the carcinoma upward to the base of the skull involves many cranial nerves, though some more frequently than others.

Histopathology

The histopathology of carcinoma of the nasopharynx shows wide variations. Some are well differentiated tumours with keratinization; others are composed of anaplastic cells without any organized arrangement and active mitoses are seen in their nuclei. In the anaplastic tumours lymphoid cells are intimately mixed from the carcinoma cells, making it difficult to differentiate them from a sarcoma.

Sarcoma

Several varieties of sarcoma occur in the nasopharynx, but they are uncommon.

Lymphosarcoma

A lymphosarcoma may be a primary tumour in the nasopharynx with, except for metastases in the regional lymph nodes, no further spread of the disease. In other patients nasopharyngeal lymphosarcoma is part of a generalized disease with tumour deposits in many tissues of the body.

In a series of necropsy cases studied were details of two patients. The first was a male patient aged 43 years. In this case, the posterior wall of the nasopharynx was replaced by a lymphosarcoma 2 cm in thickness adherent to the base of the skull. Lymphosarcoma was present in the right internal auditory meatus and the regional lymph nodes. Tumour deposits were distributed in many organs and tissues which included the skin, subcutaneous tissues, left biceps muscle, lungs, heart, mediastinal lymph nodes, common bile duct, pancreas, duodenum and kidneys. The liver was not affected.

The second case was a female patient aged 59 years. A lymphosarcoma was present in the nasopharynx with metastases in the regional lymph nodes. The patient developed infective meningitis.

Spindle cell sarcoma

In the necropsy series studied there was only one case of a spindle cell sarcoma in the nasopharynx, that of a female aged 4 years with a tumour affecting the nasopharynx, palate and base of the skull. The tumour was soft, fleshy and white and it covered most of the left lateral and posterior walls of the nasopharynx, replacing the greater part of the body of the sphenoid bone and sella turcica and displacing the pituitary gland. Laterally the tumour involved the greater wing of the sphenoid bone and the squamous portion of the temporal bone, invading the inferior surface of the temporal lobe of the left cerebral hemisphere. The left middle ear was entirely replaced by the tumour, which reached the skin and subcutaneous tissues of the left mastoid region. The foramen lacerum and optic foramen were occluded. There were no lymph node metastases. On histopathology, the appearances were those of a spindle cell sarcoma and spheroidal, stellate and strap-like cells were also present.

Rhabdomyosarcoma

Rhabdomyosarcoma is a rare tumour in the nasopharynx, usually seen in children and young adults. The tumour has a lobulated, polypoid, white, fleshy appearance and is firm in consistency. It may be sessile or pedunculated; it spreads by direct extension locally and metastases are formed in the regional lymph nodes. Spread by the bloodstream causes widespread metastases.

Histopathology shows diverse appearances, but the characteristic features include long, tubular and strap-like cells with acidophilic cytoplasm showing longitudinal and transverse striation. Cells are also present which are less well differentiated and this is the criterion of malignancy.

Salivary gland type of tumour

The subject of salivary gland type of tumours was studied by Harrison[2] based on a series of 82 cases and he gave a historical review also. He distinguished three types based on histopathology, namely mixed adenoma, cylindroma, and other adenomas. The majority of cylindromas arise in ectopic sites, possess a characteristic histopathology appearance, and occur more commonly around the foregut and upper part of the respiratory tract. They infiltrate contiguous tissues and produce metastases but progress more slowly than carcinoma. Unless these tumours are excised radically they recur locally.

In Harrison's series[2] the tumours were situated in the nasopharynx where they arise from the glands of the mucous membrane and not from ectopic salivary gland tissue. Invasion of the base of the skull may occur before distant metastases develop.

Plasma cell tumour

Plasma cell tumours have a wide distribution in the upper air passages and oral cavity; they are rarely multiple. The tumour arises in the mucous membrane of the nasopharynx and is sessile or polypoid, varying from greyish-red to dark red in colour. As it enlarges lobulation develops, but surface ulceration is uncommon.

The tumour spreads locally by invading the adjacent mucous membrane, but deep invasion of bone is uncommon. Metastases may occur in the regional and other groups of lymph nodes and in the bone marrow.

Histopathology shows masses of plasma cells which are separated by connective tissue septa. The individual cells vary in size; some are multinucleated. Mitotic figures are variable, and Russell bodies are absent. Evidence of infiltration is seen.

Chordoma

Chordoma is a very rare tumour in the nasopharynx.

This tumour arises from the remains of the notochord and is non-encapsulated, soft in consistency and gelatinous. It spreads by local infiltration of contiguous tissues; metastases are rare. The histopathology resembles the foetal notochord. There are islands and columns of vacuolated (physaliphorus) cells in a mucinous matrix.

Case record A male patient aged 38 years was referred from another country with a recurrent chordoma of the nasopharynx for which two operations of excision had been performed 3 and 2 years previously. He developed a recurrence and a rapidly increasing tetraparesis. There was a palpable tumour in the nasopharynx extending into the right side of the neck behind and below the angle of the mandible. He had a right lower motor neuron twelfth nerve palsy and a flaccid tetraparesis affecting the left limbs more than the right and a sensory level at C2. A radiogram showed destruction of the body of the 2nd cervical vertebra with forward subluxation of the cervical spine in the upper cervical region.

The patient was successfully managed and treated by a neurosurgeon who applied traction to the cervical spine with improvement of the neurological condition. A tracheostomy was necessary for respiratory difficulty. Fixation of the cervical spine was carried out by a cervical–occipital fusion and the arch of the atlas vertebra was removed. Rehabilitation resulted in excellent movements of the upper and lower extremities and the patient became fully ambulant. Radiotherapy with a tumour dose of 6000 R caused some regression of the chordoma in the nasopharynx. The patient then returned home to his country.

TUMOURS OF THE OROPHARYNX

Compared with other organs and sites of the body the oropharynx is a relatively uncommon site for the development of both benign and malignant tumours.

Benign tumour

Benign tumours are very rare in the oropharynx.

Neurilemmoma of the oropharynx

Case record   A female aged 41 years had noticed a swelling in the left side of her neck for 8 months. On examination there was a round, smooth, mobile tumour of the left tonsil displacing forward the anterior faucial pillar. The tumour was firm in consistency, not ulcerated, and continuous with the upper left cervical tumour which extended from the mastoid process to the left submandibular region and measured 6.5 × 8 cm.

Histopathology appearances were typical of a neurilemmoma with prominent cell regimentation. The capsule of the tumour contained nerve bundles.

The patient was treated with radiotherapy with a maximum tumour dose of 1800 R over 15 days. The tumour regressed completely and there was no recurrence 13 years and 10 months later.

Malignant tumours

Malignant tumours are uncommon in the oropharynx when compared with other sites in the body. Carcinoma is more frequent than the other varieties.

Carcinoma

Carcinoma of the oropharynx usually arises in the tonsil, or in the anterior or posterior pillar of the fauces.

Appearance

There are three varieties. A *malignant ulcer* is the most frequent type showing the usual characteristic features and involves the tonsil or a faucial pillar. It sometimes arises at the junction of the anterior pillar with the upper surface of the posterior third of the tongue. A *nodular tumour* is another type which has an irregular surface and projects into the lumen of the oropharynx. The base is indurated and superficial ulceration may be present. A *hard submucous tumour* is uncommon and affects the tonsil, being covered by its mucous membrane, and there is no ulceration.

Histopathology

Carcinoma of the oropharynx is a squamous cell tumour whose early appearance is the malignant transformation of the epidermis – carcinoma *in situ*. There are various degrees of differentiation. Thus the tumour is anaplastic and composed of small polyhedral and cuboidal cells with little or no organized arrangement.

The tonsil may be densely infiltrated by a squamous cell carcinoma which is largely undifferentiated, but in the deeper parts there are prickle cells without any keratinization. The nuclei may show marked hyperchromatism. In other tumours there is well-marked keratinization.

Histopathology provides evidence of spread. Deposits of tumour may be seen scattered in the surrounding areolar tissue. Tumour cells may be seen in nerve sheaths and in the lumen of the internal carotid artery, and the internal jugular vein may be invaded by tumour cells.

Methods of dissemination

Spread by direct extension   The carcinoma infiltrates the soft tissues in its vicinity to involve the lateral wall of the oropharynx including the tonsil and faucial pillars. Upward extension occurs into the nasopharynx and the base of the skull, which is penetrated later to expose the dura mater. Extension inwards gradually destroys the soft and hard palates and the uvula. The tumour spreads across the midline of the posterior wall into the structures of the opposite side, and when the posterior wall is penetrated the carcinoma infiltrates the perivertebral tissues and the bodies of the cervical vertebrae. In one patient the tumour extended through the intervertebral foramina into the extradural space where it compressed the cervical segment of the spinal cord. Downward extension occurs into the base of the tongue.

Spread by the lymphatics Metastases occur frequently in the regional lymph nodes. The lymphatic vessels of the oropharynx pass to the jugulodigastric lymph node and the lymph node lying immediately below, where metastases initially occur. There are many intercommunicating lymphatic vessels in the neck and consequently the metastases soon become more widespread. When the primary carcinoma is confined to one half of the oropharynx, the cervical lymph nodes on the same side are primarily involved, but metastases may also be present in the opposite lymph nodes. When the carcinoma has transgressed the midline, bilateral cervical lymph node metastases may be present.

Spread by the blood vessels Haematogenous metastases are not common. A carcinomatous mass was present in a bronchus in one of the author's patients, and in another a metastasis occurred in the pancreas.

A rare combination of tumours
In the author's series of cases of carcinoma of the oropharynx, one patient, a female aged 66 years with an extensive oropharyngeal carcinoma, also had seven argentaffinomas in the ileum measuring up to 1.5 cm in diameter and some were umbilicated. They were situated in the submucous tissues and penetrated through the bowel wall to the serosa.

Surgical treatment
Surgical operations for the various stages of carcinoma have been described by Raven.[3]

Case record A male patient aged 61 years was referred with an extensive carcinoma of the oropharynx which involved the left tonsil, anterior and posterior pillars of the fauces, the adjacent soft palate and the base of the tongue. The left upper deep cervical lymph nodes were enlarged.

This advanced carcinoma was considered to be unresponsive to radiotherapy, so a left partial palatoglossopharyngectomy combined with a left radical dissection of the cervical lymph nodes was performed. The defect in the wall of the oropharynx was repaired immediately with an inner mucous membrane lining reflected from the dorsolateral surface of the tongue and an outer skin cover. A temporary tracheostomy was instituted. The patient made an excellent recovery with perfect wound healing and the tracheostomy closed spontaneously (Figures 1–3).

Histopathology showed a squamous cell primary carcinoma of the oropharynx and metastases in the cervical lymph nodes.

The patient was alive and well 10 years after the operation and there was no recurrent or metastatic carcinoma.

Sarcoma
Sarcoma is rare in the oropharynx, but several varieties do occur.

Fibrosarcoma
Case record A female aged 44 years was referred with a tumour in the oropharynx discerned 2 months previously in another country when she was examined for a sore throat. There were no other symptoms except a recent burning sensation in her throat after eating food.

Examination revealed an oval tumour in the retropharyngeal tissues projecting forward into the posterior wall of the left side of the oropharynx (Figure 4). A superficial ulcer marked the site of a previous biopsy. The tumour measured 3 × 2 cm and extended upwards into the nasopharynx. Both tonsils were normal and the cervical lymph nodes were not enlarged.

The surgical technique for the excision of this tumour in a relatively inaccessible site was considered carefully, and a decision was made to use the transbuccal approach. The posterior wall of the

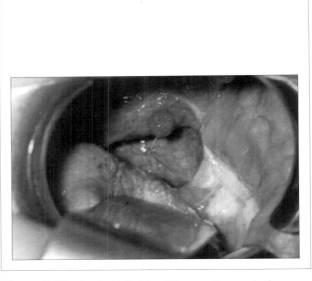

Figure 2 The healed left side of the oropharynx in the same patient

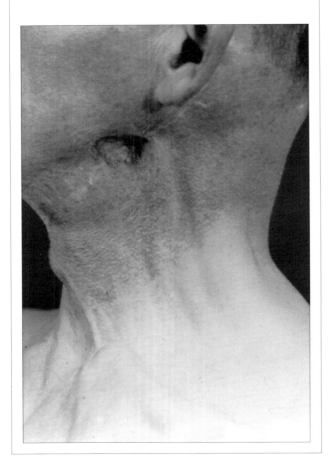

Figure 1 Male patient aged 61 years showing his healed neck after partial palatoglossopharyngectomy for an advanced squamous cell carcinoma of the left side of the oropharynx

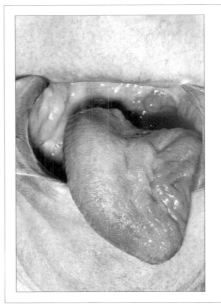

Figure 3 His functional tongue following partial palatoglossopharyngectomy

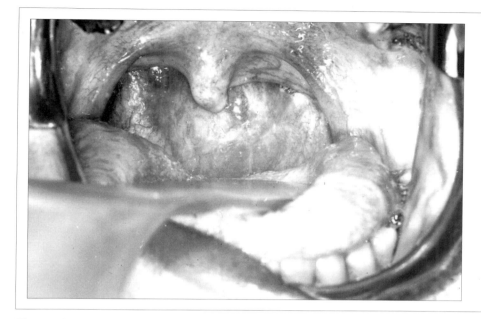

Figure 4 Female aged 44 years with a fibrosarcoma of the oropharynx causing a swelling of the posterior wall

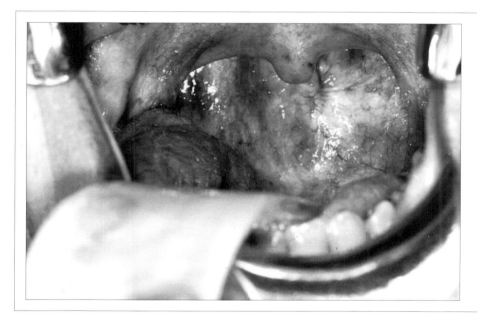

Figure 5 The healed oropharynx following transbuccal excision of the fibrosarcoma

oropharynx covering the tumour was incised longitudinally and the flaps reflected to expose the tumour. This was dissected off the anterior common ligament of the cervical vertebrae and removed. The posterior pharyngeal wall was sutured and a temporary tracheostomy instituted. The patient made an uninterrupted recovery with good healing of the oropharynx and the tracheostomy closed spontaneously (Figure 5).

A postoperative course of radiotherapy was given to the tumour site and upper deep cervical lymph nodes.

Histopathology showed the typical appearance of a fibrosarcoma.

The patient was well 26 years following the operation and there was no recurrent or metastatic tumour.

Figures 6–9 show the technique of transbuccal excision of fibrosarcoma of the oropharynx.

Reticulosarcoma

The author has had three patients with a reticulosarcoma of the oropharynx, which manifested itself primarily in the tonsil. These patients received radiotherapy. In one patient the primary tumour and regional lymph nodes disappeared and 7 months later there was no sign of the tonsil tumour and regional lymph nodes. Other groups of lymph nodes had appeared which were treated with radiotherapy and chemotherapy, but death occurred 18 months after the first treatment. Autopsy showed reticulosarcoma of the right tonsil with spread of the disease to the thoracic and coeliac lymph nodes and lung metastases.

The second patient responded well to radiotherapy, for there was no sign of local disease 3 years and 6 months later. However, he developed carcinoma of the caecum 3 years and 2 months after the radiotherapy, and an ileotransverse colostomy was

performed. The patient died during the 4th year following his initial treatment.

The third patient received radiotherapy for the reticulosarcoma of the oropharynx but he died 22 months following treatment; active local disease was present.

Histopathology appearances of reticulosarcoma of the oropharynx are of a poorly differentiated sarcoma with eosinophil leukocytes. Inflammatory changes occur around the tumour. The appearances resemble a very active undifferentiated anaplastic carcinoma (Figure 10).

Lymphosarcoma

This disease may commence in the tonsil, which becomes enlarged and red in colour, and sometimes a superficial ulcer occurs. Both tonsils may be affected simultaneously. The disease spreads through the lymphatics to the cervical lymph nodes, followed by distant lymph nodes including the axillary, intrathoracic, coeliac axis, pelvic and inguinal groups. There may be cutaneous deposits of lymphosarcoma.

In other patients the tonsil is affected as part of generalized lymphosarcoma disease where many organs and tissues are affected including the spleen, liver, stomach, pancreas, intestine, peritoneum, diaphragm, lungs, pericardium and many groups of lymph nodes. This variety of the disease was present in three cases studied at autopsy.

Histopathology reveals a thin layer of squamous epithelium and connective tissue overlying the tumour, composed of round cells which resemble mature lymphocytes or immature lymphocytes with various degrees of anaplasia. The cells are based mainly on a very delicate connective tissue reticulum.

Anaplastic carcinoma (lymphoepithelioma)

The author had a patient with this variety of tumour, known as lymphoepithelioma. The tumour involved

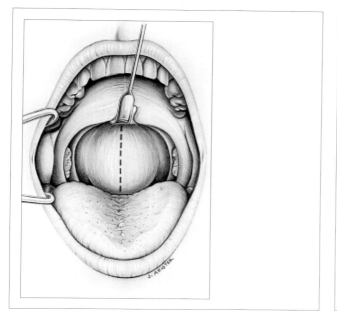

Figure 6 The transbuccal operation for excision of a fibrosarcoma: the soft palate is retracted upwards and a longitudinal incision (dotted line) is made over the tumour

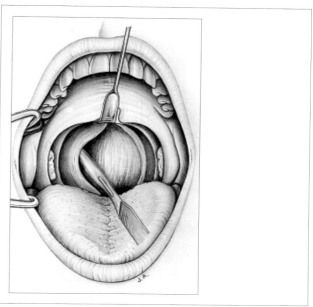

Figure 7 The posterior wall of the oropharynx is reflected off the tumour

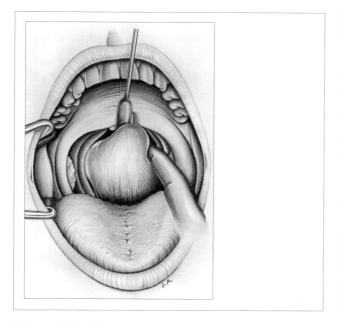

Figure 8 The fibrosarcoma is removed from its bed, which includes the anterior common ligament of the cervical vertebrae

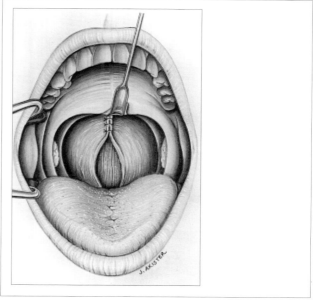

Figure 9 The incision in the posterior wall of the oropharynx is sutured with interrupted sutures of catgut, and a temporary tracheostomy is formed

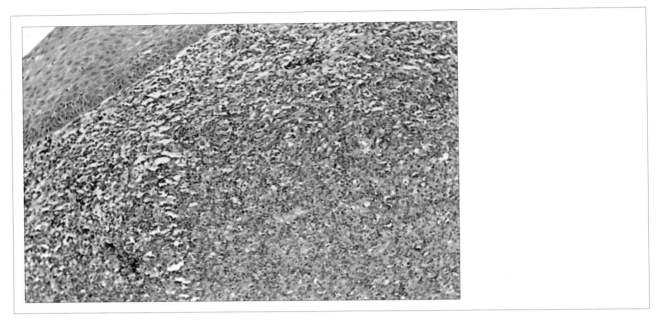

Figure 10 Histopathology appearance of a reticulosarcoma of the tonsil

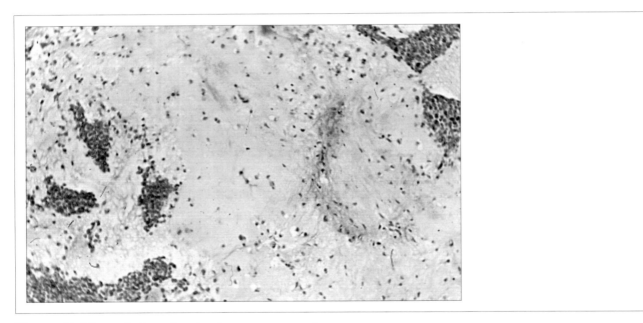

Figure 11 Histopathology showing the appearance of a mixed salivary gland type of tumour with the epithelial and mucoid areas

the right tonsillar area and was treated with radiotherapy to the local disease (maximal tumour dose 4600 R) and to the right cervical lymph nodes (maximal tumour dose 4000 R in 43 days). There was complete regression of the tumour and 16 years and 6 months later there was no sign of disease.

Mixed salivary gland tumour

Tumours of the mixed salivary gland variety are not common and arise in the tonsil or fauces causing a unilateral swelling, which may be large, in the oropharynx. The tumour frequently extends into the nasopharynx, deforming the palate, and it may bulge laterally into the neck producing a swelling in the region of the angle of the mandible. The surface of a larger tumour is frequently ulcerated superficially. Metastases may occur in the regional cervical lymph nodes.

The primary tumour and regional lymph nodes are excised when the disease is operable. A course of postoperative radiotherapy may be indicated by the extent of the tumour.

Recurrent tumour may occur as shown in the following example. A mixed salivary gland tumour in the oropharynx was partially excised; complete excision was not possible because of two deep tumour prolongations. Postoperative radiotherapy was given at a tumour dose of 5000 R in 50 days. The patient made good progress, but a recurrent tumour developed 5 years and 4 months later, and this was excised. A second recurrent tumour was excised another 5 years and 10 months later and a third recurrent tumour in the right side of the soft palate was excised another 9 years and 11 months later.

Figure 11 shows the histopathological appearance of a mixed salivary gland tumour.

Plasma cell tumour

Plasma cell tumour occurs in the nasopharynx, and its features have been described earlier in this chapter. It also occurs in the oropharynx.

The tumour spreads by direct extension, by the lymphatics to the regional and other groups of lymph nodes and by the bloodstream.

Malignant melanoma

This very malignant tumour rarely occurs in the oropharynx. In the author's series of cases of tumours of the pharynx there was only one such patient. This was a male patient aged 53 years with a malignant melanoma affecting the right tonsil. Extensive tumour dissemination had occurred causing metastases in the regional cervical lymph nodes and in many viscera.

Malignant melanoma occurring in a structure covered by mucous membrane is particularly malignant.

TUMOURS OF THE HYPOPHARYNX

Carcinoma

Primary carcinoma is the most common tumour in the hypopharynx and this is the main subject of this section. The diagnosis of these malignant tumours is made today in a much earlier stage of development than several decades ago and the examples shown here of extensive and advanced carcinomas are rarely seen at the present time. In earlier years the tumour often extended from the cervical oesophagus to the oropharynx and converted the hypopharynx into a solid carcinomatous tube.

The carcinoma rises in different parts of the hypopharynx; in the author's experience the pyriform fossa is the most common site followed by the postcricoid region. The tumour may arise less often in the posterior wall, epiglottis, and the glosso-epiglottic and aryepiglottic folds.

Appearance

Described here are five varieties. The common type

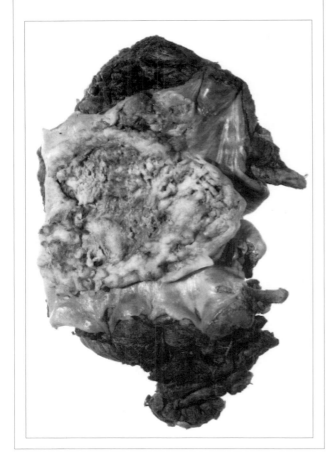

Figure 12 A carcinoma of the hypopharynx involving the postcricoid region, removed by laryngo-oesophagopharyngectomy

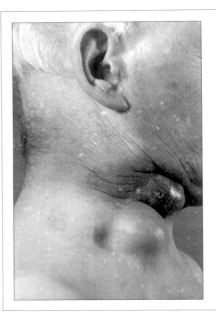

Figure 13 Male patient with an advanced carcinoma in the pyriform fossa of the hypopharynx spreading by direct extension to ulcerate the skin of the neck and by the lymphatics to form lymph node metastases

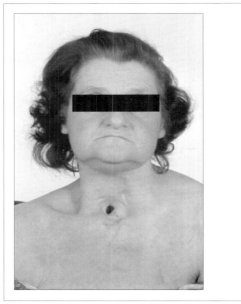

Figure 14 Patient with an extensive squamous cell carcinoma of the hypopharynx and cervical oesophagus after laryngo-oesophagopharyngectomy with reconstruction of the hypopharynx and cervical oesophagus

is a *malignant ulcer* with the usual features including a hard proliferative edge. A *flat plaque* is less frequent and forms a raised tumour in the pharyngeal wall with a smooth surface and without ulceration. A *nodular tumour* projects into the lumen of the hypopharynx and has an irregular surface, superficially ulcerated, and an indurated base. A *pedunculated tumour* is uncommon; it arises by a stalk from a localized area of pharyngeal wall and the main part is irregular and ulcerated on the surface. In several of the author's patients there was solid filling of the hypopharynx with *diffuse tumour infiltration* of the whole extent of the wall and completely filling its lumen. An illustration is shown in Figure 12 of a specimen removed by the operation of laryngo-oesophagopharyngectomy.

Histopathology

Carcinoma of the hypopharynx is usually a squamous cell tumour which is often well differentiated, and various degrees of keratinization are present. Sometimes the tumour is composed of anaplastic cells arranged in solid sheets of variable size and showing active mitosis. In some tumours the cells are atypical and tend to form an alveolar arrangement. The submucous tissues may be involved for considerable distances beyond the macroscopic edge of the tumour and these extensions may show more differentiated cells, keratinization and cell nests. In addition there may be considerable invasion of the mucous glands.

There are variations in histology appearances. For example, one part of the tumour may be anaplastic and another area well differentiated. Oedema of some cells is also seen. The mucous membrane in the vicinity of a carcinoma may show carcinoma *in situ* changes.

Carcinoma cells can be demonstrated in the submucosal lymphatics beyond the edge of the main tumour and in the lymphatics of different parts of the hypopharynx and larynx including the aryepiglottic fold, the ventricle and the vocal cords. They are seen in the perineural lymphatics of the large trunks and in the lumen of the internal jugular vein. They are also found along the sarcolemma of muscles.

Methods of dissemination

Spread by direct extension The carcinoma increases in size and in depth in the wall of the hypopharynx, and structures beyond are invaded (Figure 13). The disease spreads upwards into the oropharynx to involve the base of the tongue, tonsils and faucial pillars and the wall. Sometimes the tumour spreads into the nasopharynx. Downward extension into the cervical oesophagus is frequent. Anteriorly the carcinoma infiltrates the larynx, and the wall of the trachea may be penetrated. The tumour spreads laterally through the pharyngeal wall into neighbouring structures. The lateral lobes of the thyroid gland are invaded frequently. Invasion of the carotid sheath and great blood vessels of the neck may cause fatal haemorrhage. Lateral extension sometimes paralyses the recurrent laryngeal nerve and the neck muscles may be infiltrated. Posteriorly the carcinoma penetrates through the pharyngeal wall into the connective tissue, ligaments and bodies of the cervical vertebrae. The thyroid and cricoid cartilages are invaded infrequently.

Spread by the lymphatics Metastases are frequent and may be extensive in the regional lymph nodes (Figure 13). Initially, metastases form in the group of cervical lymph nodes receiving lymph from the hypopharynx through the supraglottic pedicle; these lie near the internal jugular vein between the posterior belly of the digastric and the anterior belly of the omohyoid muscles. A carcinoma anywhere in the hypopharynx can metastasize to these lymph nodes and when it is limited to one half of the hypopharynx, the lymph nodes in both sides of the neck may be affected. These lymph nodes draining lymph from the supraglottic pedicle communicate with the lymph nodes lying along the spinal accessory nerve as far as the anterior border of the trapezius muscle, and with lymph nodes below the omohyoid muscle as far as the supraclavicular region. Metastases can also pass from the lymph nodes in one side of the neck to those in the opposite side.

A carcinoma in the postcricoid region and cervical oesophagus metastasizes to the group of lymph nodes lying along the recurrent laryngeal nerve in one or both sides of the neck. When the tumour infiltrates the larynx, metastases may be found in the prelaryngeal and pretracheal lymph nodes in addition to the perithyroidean lymphatics in the thyroid gland capsule. When the carcinoma has invaded the lymphatic system, metastases may be found in lymph nodes far from the primary tumour, including prevertebral and mediastinal nodes, those along the lesser curvature of the stomach and those in the pancreas and in the portal fissure of the liver.

Spread by the blood vessels Direct invasion of the internal jugular vein may occur and it is likely that smaller blood vessels are affected similarly causing metastases in other parts of the body. They occur most often in the lung involving a bronchus or the parenchyma. Metastases have been seen in the myocardium and liver.

Treatment

The majority of the author's patients had advanced carcinoma of the hypopharynx which had frequently infiltrated into the cervical oesophagus, larynx, trachea and thyroid gland. In 47% of the patients there were histologically-proven carcinoma metastases in the cervical lymph nodes. The patients suffered severely from dysphagia, dyspnoea and stridor.

In some patients a palliative gastrostomy or tracheostomy had already been performed in other clinics. Some of the patients had been pronounced untreatable and, with the aid of sedatives, awaited death. Others had undergone radiotherapy of maximum tumour dosage which failed to control the disease, and the severe radiation effects in the skin and other tissues of the neck caused additional problems for surgical treatment.

A laryngo-oesophagopharyngectomy was performed with a radical dissection of the cervical lymph nodes when metastases were present. Normal deglutition was restored by reconstruction of the hypopharynx and cervical oesophagus with a whole-thickness skin tube, and a permanent tracheostomy was established which relieved the respiratory difficulties. This two-stage major procedure was carried out for those patients considered suitable after careful investigations were done.

Case record A female patient had an extensive carcinoma of the hypopharynx and cervical oesophagus which caused considerable dysphagia. A laryngo-oesophagopharyngectomy was performed as a two-stage operation with reconstruction of the hypopharynx and cervical oesophagus with whole-thickness skin flaps. A permanent tracheostomy was instituted and normal deglutition was restored. Histopathology showed a squamous cell carcinoma. The patient was alive 22 years after the operation and there was no recurrent or metastatic disease (Figure 14).

Case record A male patient had an extensive carcinoma of the hypopharynx uncontrolled by a full tumour dosage of radiotherapy. Emergency tracheostomy had been necessary for severe dyspnoea. Severe radiation changes were present in the neck skin with extensive dermatitis (Figure 15). Laryngo-oesophagopharyngectomy was performed and reconstruction of the new hypopharynx and cervical oesophagus was done in multiple stages. A permanent tracheostomy was instituted.

Histopathology showed anaplastic ulcerating carcinoma occupying the right pyriform fossa extending to involve the true and false vocal cords in the larynx. Metastases were present in the cervical lymph nodes.

Postoperative healing was good (Figure 16) and the patient had perfect deglutition, as shown on X-ray (Figure 17). He returned to work and had no recurrent carcinoma in his neck. He died 12 years and 6 months later from bronchogenic carcinoma.

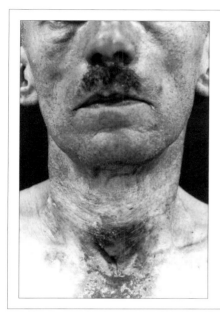

Figure 15 A male patient with an extensive anaplastic ulcerating carcinoma of the hypopharynx uncontrolled by full tumour dosage of radiotherapy. Emergency tracheostomy had been necessary for severe dyspnoea. Severe radiation changes were present in the neck skin with extensive dermatitis

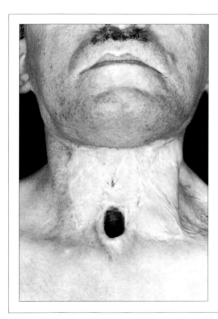

Figure 16 The same patient as in Figure 15 showing the healed neck following laryngo-oesophagopharyngectomy and reconstruction of the hypopharynx and cervical oesophagus

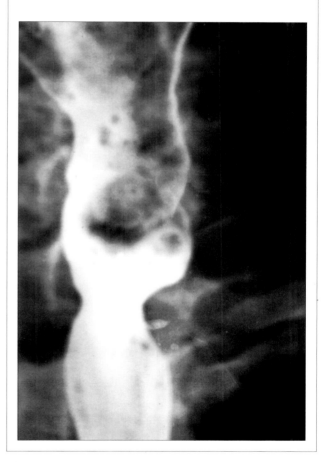

Figure 17 The same patient as in Figure 16 showing the radiograph with a barium swallow of the new skin hypopharynx and its junction with the oesophagus. Perfect deglutition was achieved

59

Radiation carcinoma of the hypopharynx

Carcinoma of the hypopharynx caused by radiotherapy for a benign condition many years previously is rare, but a number of cases have been reported in the literature in patients who had received radiotherapy for thyrotoxicosis or tuberculous cervical adenitis an average of 25 years earlier[4]. The following case record was published by Raven and Levison[5].

Case record A female aged 46 years had been treated with radiotherapy for thyrotoxicosis 23 years earlier. The exact dosage is not known but it was calculated from available data that the pharynx had received a dose of 10 000 R ± 10% where the carcinoma subsequently occurred. Over a period of 8 months the patient had experienced increasing dysphagia with considerable food regurgitation. For 2 weeks she had had dyspnoea and voice huskiness.

Examination showed mild exophthalmos, dyspnoea and stridor. There was a wide band of telangiectasis of the skin over the anterolateral part of the neck with thickness, scarring and loss of elasticity. The hypopharynx and larynx were expanded laterally, but were mobile; the thyroid gland was indurated and the cervical lymph nodes were enlarged. Pharyngoscopy revealed a postcricoid carcinoma, confirmed by biopsy and histopathology.

A gastrostomy was instituted to build up the patient's general condition to undergo laryngo-oesophagopharyngectomy. One month later the neck was explored with this objective, but the carcinoma proved inoperable, having infiltrated the retropharyngeal tissues and become necrotic. A tracheostomy was instituted. The patient died 4 months later.

Radiotherapy was given many years ago when there were no accurate methods of estimating dosage, nor any recognized unit of dosage. New methods of radiotherapy are now used with careful control of dosage so that the skin and other tissues are not damaged.

Squamous carcinoma associated with polypoid pseudosarcoma

This is a rare tumour in the hypopharynx; the author has experience of only one patient. There was a short history of voice hoarseness and dysphagia in a male aged 63 years. Later dyspnoea and stridor developed, and some weight loss. Examination revealed a large irregular tumour arising in the medial wall of the right pyriform fossa and involving the whole right arytenoid, from which is extended to cover most of the glottis. Radiotherapy was given with a maximum tumour dose of 6500 R and 4840 R to the lymph node area in 63 days with complete regression. The patient died 3 years later from cerebral thrombosis. There was no recurrent tumour.

Histopathology showed a bulky tumour with little tendency to infiltrate the pharyngeal wall. Microscopy showed scattered foci of keratinizing squamous carcinoma, but the main tumour bulk was composed of dense collagenous fibrous tissue diffusely infiltrated with large irregular cells lying singly or in small clusters (Figure 18). Many cells had bizarre giant hyperchromatic nuclei and eosinophilic cytoplasm which was vacuolated, or contained numerous hyaline droplets. There were considerable numbers of mitotic figures, many being abnormal. The surface was covered partly by a layer of stratified squamous epithelium, and partly by non-specific granulation tissue containing many polymorphs. Some of the large stromal cells had polymorphs within their cytoplasm. This was a squamous carcinoma associated with polypoid pseudosarcoma.

Rhabdomyosarcoma

Rhabdomyosarcoma of the hypopharynx is a very malignant tumour and forms widespread metastases.

Case record A female aged 36 years had experienced a 'cold' 5 weeks previously, followed by voice hoarseness, cough and increasing dyspnoea which necessitated a tracheostomy. Examination showed fixation of the right half of the larynx; there was an ulcer affecting almost the whole upper part of the right pyriform fossa involving the medial and lateral walls and the floor. There were two enlarged cervical lymph nodes. She was treated with radiotherapy (telecobalt) with a maximum tumour dose of 6585 R in 52 days. Following radiotherapy a pharyng-olaryngectomy with total thyroidectomy and right radical lymph node block dissection was performed.

Histopathology showed the tumour to be composed of loosely arranged large irregular cells with vesicular nuclei and abundant cytoplasm; some cells were spherical and others were elongated and fusiform. There was abundant and highly vascular stroma. No cross striations were demonstrated, but the appearances were suggestive of a rhabdomyosarcoma.

The patient died 4 months after the operation with multiple metastases

Case record A male aged 62 years had experienced a sore throat and laryngitis 12 months previously, followed 8 months later by intermittent voice hoarseness, dysphagia and cough. Examination revealed thickening of the right half of the larynx and hypopharynx and a small lymph node in the right upper deep cervical group draining the supraglottic lymphatic pedicle. A tumour filled the right pyriform fossa. He was given pre-operative radiotherapy with a maximum tumour dose of 5450 R in 43 days. This was followed by laryngo-oesophagopharyngectomy in two stages. The patient was alive with pulmonary metastases 15 months after the operation; there was no local neck recurrence; the patient swallowed perfectly and his general condition was good.

The pathology report described the specimen as a tumour filling the right pyriform fossa 4 × 4.5 cm with ulceration 3.5 × 1.5 cm over the right lateral aspect. The tumour had grown between the thyroid cartilage and laryngeal mucosa, had destroyed the cricoid cartilage and extended to the left arytenoid cartilage.

Except for the ulcerated area, the pharyngeal mucosa was remarkably mobile over the yellow tumour nodules visible through it. The thyroid gland was normal.

Histopathology of the specimen showed a pleomorphic sarcoma structure with large strap-shaped and spindle cells, bizarre and multinucleate types (Figure 19). In the spindle cells, faint horizontal striations were seen in the cytoplasm and there was a pericellular reticulum pattern. The tumour was a poorly differentiated rhabdomyosarcoma. The regional lymph nodes were free of metastases.

Spread of the disease
The tumour spreads through the bloodstream; the male patient had radiological signs of pulmonary metastases 2 months after the operation. The female patient, at autopsy, had metastases in the lungs, liver, pancreas and kidney; in addition, bilateral ovarian teratoma was found.

Plasma cell tumour
A plasma cell tumour is rare in the hypopharynx; it also occurs in the nasopharynx and oropharynx and in the upper air passages, tongue, floor of the mouth, nose and accessory air sinuses. Rarely multiple tumours are present.

A plasma cell tumour is sessile or polypoid and arises in the mucous membrane of the organ affected. As it enlarges, the tumour becomes lobulated; surface ulceration is uncommon.

Methods of spread
By direct extension The tumour spreads locally by invading the adjacent mucous membrane of the hypopharynx, but deep invasion in the bone and cartilage is uncommon.

By the lymphatics Metastases are formed in the regional lymph nodes and other groups of lymph nodes.

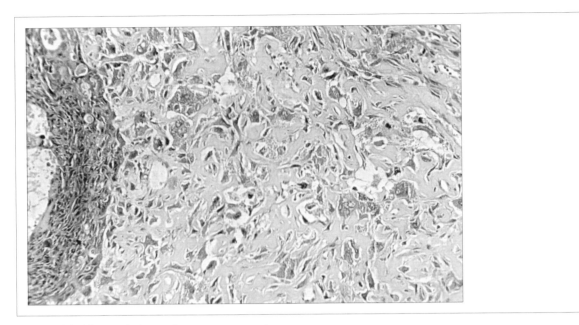

Figure 18 Histopathology of a squamous carcinoma associated with polypoid pseudosarcoma of the hypopharynx. The section shows both the carcinomatous and the pseudosarcomatous components (H & E low magnification)

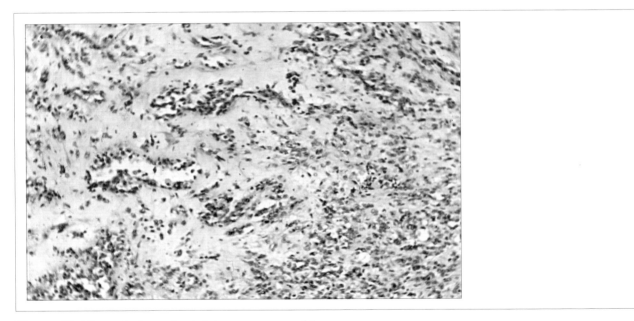

Figure 19 Histopathology of a rhabdomyosarcoma of the hypopharynx. The section shows long strap-like cells widely separated by oedema (H & E low magnification)

By the blood vessels Metastases are found in the bone marrow of one or more bones.

Histopathology
The tumour is composed of masses of plasma cells separated by connective tissue septa. The individual cells vary in size and some are multinucleated; mitotic figures are variable. There is evidence of local infiltration.

Carcinoma of the hypopharynx associated with another primary carcinoma
Clinical and autopsy cases where a carcinoma of the hypopharynx either preceded or followed a primary carcinoma in another organ have been recorded by Raven[6]. These other associations were primary carcinoma of the colon, tongue, breast, rectum, skin and stomach.

REFERENCES

1. Wilson, C. P. (1951). The approach to the nasopharynx. *Proc. Roy. Soc. Med.*, **44**, 353–8
2. Harrison, K. (1956). Study of ectopic mixed salivary tumours (Hunterian lecture). *Ann. Roy. Coll. Surg. Engl.*, **18**, 99–122
3. Raven, R. W. (1958). *Cancer of the Pharynx, Larynx and Oesophagus and its Surgical Treatment*, pp. 74–92. (London: Butterworth & Co.)
4. Raven, R. W. (1958). *Cancer of the Pharynx, Larynx and Oesophagus and its Surgical Treatment*, Ch. 4. (London: Butterworth & Co.)
5. Raven, R. W. and Levison, V. B. (1954). Radiation cancer of pharynx. *Lancet*, **2**, 683–4
6. Raven, R. W. (1958). *Cancer of the Pharynx, Larynx and Oesophagus and its Surgical Treatment*, pp. 103–4. (London: Butterworth & Co.)

5

Tumours of the oesophagus

THE PATERSON–KELLY SYNDROME

The Paterson–Kelly syndrome is regarded as a precursor condition of carcinoma of the mouth, pharynx (especially the postcricoid region) and oesophagus in females. Kelly[1] described the symptoms in a group of female patients, consisting of dysphagia with frequent arrest of food at the oesophageal entrance, regurgitation of liquids, and nervousness when eating. Sometimes there was a long history of anaemia, dysphagia or impaired general health. In some patients the tongue was smooth and devoid of papillae, the mucous membrane of the mouth and pharynx had a dry, waxy appearance and fissures were present at the angles of the mouth. In one patient there was a circular membranous web which reduced the oesophageal entrance to about 5 mm in diameter; when this was ruptured the symptoms were relieved.

Paterson[2] drew attention to the association of spasmodic dysphagia with superficial glossitis confined to females. He described the thinness of the mucous membrane over the cricoid cartilage which cracks with the slightest pressure due to loss of resilience, permitting the cricoid cartilage to tilt forward, thus allowing a clear view of the introitus. He also stated that malignant disease supervened not infrequently in the mouth and gullet and this occurred too often to be a coincidence.

Vinson[3] reported a series of 69 cases, 57 females and 12 males. Their characteristic symptoms were sudden onset of dysphagia and the development of secondary anaemia; in 12 patients splenomegaly, usually marked, was present. The duration of symptoms varied from 1 month to 25 years; the anaemia was more common in patients having long-standing dysphagia.

Case record A female aged 60 years had had dysphagia for 3 years and was found to have anaemia which was treated with iron therapy. One year after the dysphagia had commenced, the Paterson–Kelly syndrome had been diagnosed with the typical lesions, including slight webbing of the oesophagus. The patient had improved with treatment until 4 months previously when she developed soreness of her throat.

Examination revealed a carcinoma in the hypopharynx, involving the left pyriform fossa and spreading to the left arytenoid cartilage and aryepiglottic fold. Metastases were present in the left upper deep cervical lymph nodes. Biopsy and histopathology showed that the primary tumour was a squamous cell carcinoma.

Case record A female aged 33 years had had a 'sensitive throat' following diphtheria at the age of 9 years. Dysphagia had then been experienced for 15 years and had been worse for the previous 6 months.

Examination revealed a large carcinoma in the hypopharynx extending from the left pyriform fossa to the left arytenoid cartilage. Bilateral cervical lymph node metastases were present. Biopsy and histopathology showed that the primary tumour was a keratinizing squamous cell carcinoma.

Case record A female aged 37 years had received treatment for anaemia for 9 years; dysphagia had developed during the previous 6 months.

Examination revealed atrophic changes in the mucous membrane of the tongue and spoon-shaped finger-nails. A carcinoma was seen in the hypopharynx involving the postcricoid region. Biopsy and histopathology showed that the primary tumour was an infiltrating, keratinizing squamous cell carcinoma.

It will be noted that these patients were females aged from 33 to 67 years with an average age of 50.2 years. Dysphagia was experienced for 2 months to 15 years, with an average period of 5 years and 7 months. Not every patient shows all the features of this syndrome; glossitis, spoon-shaped finger-nails and splenomegaly may be absent.

The stricture at the pharyngo-oesophageal junction can be severe in patients with the Paterson–Kelly syndrome. The stricture may be impassable and excision of the pharyngo-oesophageal junction and pharyngo-oesophageal anastomosis may have to be performed.

CARCINOMA

A primary carcinoma, which is usually squamous cell in type, is the most common tumour that occurs in the oesophagus. Macroscopically there are four varieties. A *papilliferous carcinoma* is a bulky tumour which projects into and may fill the oesophageal lumen. It is friable; superficial ulceration may be present and the base is indurated. A *fibrocarcinoma* has a large quantity of fibrous tissue which causes hardness on palpation. This variety usually affects a short oesophageal segment, 2.5–5 cm. This carcinoma remains mobile longer than the papilliferous variety and causes a severe stricture with little or no ulceration. A *carcinomatous ulcer* develops in the oesophageal wall having the usual features of malignancy and causing considerable induration in the surrounding tissues. A *plaque carcinoma* forms a flat tumour, slightly raised, which develops in the oesophageal mucous membrane. It is smooth and the deeper layers of the wall of the oesophagus are little affected.

Histopathology of the majority is that of a squamous cell carcinoma, resembling those found in the mouth and pharynx. There are various degrees of differentiation, from the cornifying tumours to the structureless anaplastic tumours without epidermoid characteristics.

ADENOCARCINOMA

An adenocarcinoma occurs infrequently in the oesophagus. It may arise from the islets of gastric mucosa which are found frequently in the oesophageal mucous membrane, especially in its upper third. This tumour also arises from the oesophageal glands.

Methods of spread
Carcinoma of the oesophagus spreads by the three usual methods.

Direct extension Longitudinal spread occurs in the submucous tissues so that islets of carcinoma are found at various distances from the main tumour; these usually cannot be seen on oesophagoscopy or detected by palpation at operation. Extension downward into the stomach wall is not common, but upward extension occurs into the hypopharynx. There is lateral extension through the coats of the oesophagus and when the muscular coat is penetrated, further extension occurs into the peri-oesophageal tissues and neighbouring organs and tissues.

A carcinoma of the cervical oesophagus spreads into the thyroid gland and other neck tissues. In the upper third of the oesophagus the carcinoma invades the trachea and large blood vessels at the thoracic inlet. In the middle third, the vena azygos major, thoracic duct, aorta and the structures in the pulmonary hila are infiltrated; the lung may also be involved. In the lower third, the anterior part of the diaphragm is often invaded and the pericardium may be affected. Posteriorly, at any level the carcinoma can extend into the vertebral bodies.

Spread by the lymphatics   Metastases occur in the regional lymph nodes which drain different oesophageal segments. Carcinoma in the cervical segment forms metastases in the lymph nodes, usually three on each side, lying along the recurrent laryngeal nerves at the thoracic inlet. The lower deep cervical nodes in relation to the carotid sheath may also be involved. Carcinomas in the upper and lower thoracic segments form metastases in the lower paratracheal and posterior mediastinal group in close proximity to the oesophagus. There are lymphatic connections between the lower thoracic group and the intertracheobronchial and pretracheal lymph nodes, where metastases may occur later.

Efferent lymphatics connect the posterior mediastinal lymph nodes with the thoracic duct which is an additional route for dissemination.

The carcinoma spreads from the lower thoracic segment and oesophagogastric region into the pericardial, upper and lower left gastric groups of lymph nodes and finally into the lymph nodes around the coeliac axis artery.

Spread by the blood vessels   Haematogenous metastases are uncommon until the late stages of the disease. The carcinoma invades the vena azygos major and other veins to cause further spread in the venous system. Metastases occur in the usual sites including the liver, lungs, bones, brain, kidneys, adrenals and subcutaneous tissues.

ABNORMALITIES OF THE OESOPHAGUS AND CARCINOMA

Carcinoma sometimes develops in the oesophagus which is already abnormal, and the number of these cases reported suggests that this association is not fortuitous.

Hiatus hernia and carcinoma

Case record   A female aged 59 years gave a history of gastric ulcer for 20 years; she had experienced discomfort on swallowing for 2 years and retrosternal pain and dysphagia for 4 months. She also had achlorhydria and pernicious anaemia. Radiology showed a stricture and an ulcer in the middle of the oesophagus, disordered peristalsis, a shortened oesophagus and a partial thoracic stomach. Thoracotomy revealed a hard tumour, considered to be a carcinoma, 1.75 cm long in the middle third of the oesophagus.

Case record   A male aged 74 years gave a history of increasing dysphagia for 4 months; he had been examined radiologically at another hospital for dysphagia 4 years previously. Radiological examination now showed a malignant stricture 5 cm long involving the lower end of the oesophagus, associated with a partial thoracic stomach. A partial oesophagogastrectomy was performed.

The specimen showed an ulcerating carcinoma 3.2 cm long in the medial wall of the oesophagus, almost encircling the wall for about 2.5 cm, and extending into the stomach for 0.7 cm beyond the oesophagogastric junction. Several enlarged lymph nodes were present. Histopathology showed a well differentiated tubular and partly mucoid adenocarcinoma infiltrating through all the coats into the surrounding fat. From a total of seven cardiac lymph nodes four contained metastases; an early metastasis was present in an upper para-oesophageal lymph node; no metastasis was present in a paracardiac lymph node. The patient died 18 months later.

Congenital shortened oesophagus and carcinoma

A carcinoma may develop in the lower end of the short oesophagus or in the thoracic stomach (see also Chapter 6).

Case record   A male aged 58 years had had indigestion for several years and recurrent attacks of haematemesis for 6 weeks. Radiological examination showed a short oesophagus, a partial thoracic stomach and an organic stricture at the lower end of the oesophagus. There was some oesophageal dilatation and reversed peristalsis. A partial oesophagogastrectomy was performed. The specimen showed a carcinomatous ulcer 2.5 cm in diameter in a thoracic stomach, situated below and to the left of the cardiac orifice. No enlarged lymph nodes were present. Histopathology showed a well differentiated columnar cell adenocarcinoma of gastric origin.

Case record   A male aged 65 years had experienced dysphagia, regurgitation and chest pain for 3 months. Radiological examination showed an irregular area in a thoracic stomach with some oesophageal obstruction at the upper end of the irregularity. A partial oesophagogastrectomy was performed. The specimen showed an extensive carcinomatous ulcer in the thoracic stomach extending into the oesophagus.

Histopathology showed a columnar cell adenocarcinoma derived from the glands of the gastric mucosa. Many parts of the malignant parenchyma were well differentiated and composed of solid columns of polyhedral cells. In other areas there were 'signet ring' forms. There were multiple zones of necrosis and calcarious deposition. Tissue from the upper extremity of the specimen showed that the normal oesophageal mucosa ended abruptly in continuity with the gastric mucosa. The latter had become malignant as far as the oesophagogastric junction and had undermined the squamous epithelium of the oesophagus, which showed oedema but no malignant change. At a deeper level in the stomach wall, the adenocarcinoma had undergone secondary squamous metaplasia.

Cardiospasm associated with carcinoma

Several cases with this condition have been reported in the literature, but it is very uncommon.

RARE TUMOURS OF THE OESOPHAGUS

Adenoid cystic carcinoma or cylindroma

A cylindroma is a rare tumour in the oesophagus. It progresses at a slower rate than the usual carcinoma and infiltrates contiguous tissues. Metastases may occur in the regional lymph nodes, lungs and bone.

Case record   A male aged 62 years had noticed something sticking in his throat 2 months earlier. Oesophagoscopy showed a fungating tumour in the oesophagus situated 25 cm from the gum which apparently arose from the left lateral wall. Biopsy was performed for histopathology, which showed that the lamina propria beneath the squamous epithelium was occupied and infiltrated by a carcinoma which in many areas was an undifferentiated polygonal cell carcinoma. No definite squamous traits could be seen and in some fields the pattern was reminiscent of an adenoid cystic carcinoma or cylindroma (Figure 1). This feature, together with the presence of an occasional mucin-secreting cell, suggested an oesophageal carcinoma of mucous gland origin.

The patient was treated with a full course of radiotherapy to the tumour, with a maximum tumour dose of 6413 R. He was well 15 months following this treatment.

Adenocanthoma

Adenocanthoma is a rare tumour in the oesophagus.

Case record A male patient aged 75 years had experienced dyspepsia for 8 months before consultation. During the previous 2 months anorexia and dysphagia had developed and for 5 weeks epigastric pain had occurred 1 hour after food. A partial oesophagogastrectomy was performed through a right thoracotomy following mobilization of the stomach through a separate upper abdominal incision. The tumour involved the middle third of the oesophagus and plaques of tumour were seen in the pleura.

The specimen consisted of an oesophageal segment 12 cm long which was grossly distorted and replaced by a tumour. The tumour was solid, yellow-white, and at one end it surrounded a lymph node forming a tumour measuring 4.5 × 4 × 2 cm.

On histopathology, the structure was that of a mixed keratinizing squamous cell and adenocarcinomatous tumour — adenocanthoma — which penetrated the entire thickness of the oesophageal wall (Figures 2 and 3). Many thin-walled blood vessels were seen to be surrounded by tumour masses and there were haemorrhages in some areas, but no indisputable evidence of vascular invasion. The lymph node showed tumour invasion.

Squamous cell carcinoma with pseudosarcomatous reaction

This is a rare tumour of the oesophagus.

Case record A male aged 70 years had undergone an abdominoperineal excision of the rectum for carcinoma at age 67 years. For 2 months he had had increasing dysphagia with coughing attacks after taking fluids, and weight loss of 21 lb. There was no sign of recurrent rectal carcinoma. A partial oesophagogastrectomy with an oesophagogastric anastomosis was performed through a right thoractomy after preliminary mobilization of the stomach through an upper abdominal incision. At operation a tumour was found in the lower third of the oesophagus adherent to the pleura.

The specimen showed a malignant stricture in the lower third of the oesophagus 5 cm long. Histopathology showed the tumour to be a moderately well differentiated keratinizing oesophageal carcinoma with *in situ* changes in the mucosa. The stroma in the superficial polypoid portion of the tumour showed the pleomorphic, giant cell pattern seen in association with the pedunculated oesophageal squamous carcinoma — the pseudosarcomatous reaction.

The patient was well 3 months after the operation.

Sarcoma

Several varieties of sarcoma occur in the oesophagus, but they are uncommon and the patients affected are usually in a younger age group than those with carcinoma.

Malignant melanoma

Primary malignant melanoma is very rare in the oesophagus and exact criteria are necessary to establish the diagnosis. A case report was published by Raven and Dawson[4], who described the pathological and clinical features and tabulated the cases reported in the literature up to that date.

Case record A female aged 52 years had experienced discomfort across the anterior chest and lower dorsal region of the back when eating food, so she had become afraid to eat. These symptoms had been present for several months. There was soreness in the upper epigastrium, but no dysphagia; a sensation of 'something like a lump of cotton wool' was felt in the gullet. There was no nausea, vomiting or food regurgitation, but there was excessive salivation. These

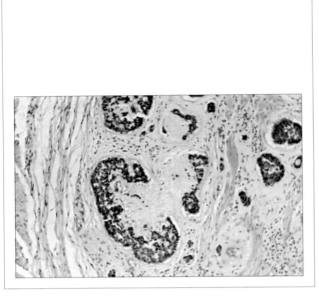

Figure 1 Histopathology of an adenoid cystic carcinoma – cylindroma – of the oesophagus. The section shows the cribriform pattern which is typical of this type of tumour (H & E)

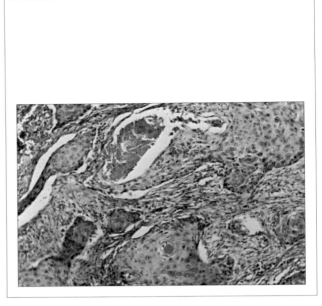

Figure 2 Adenocanthoma of the oesophagus in a male aged 75 years. Histopathology shows the keratinizing squamous cell part of the tumour (H & E)

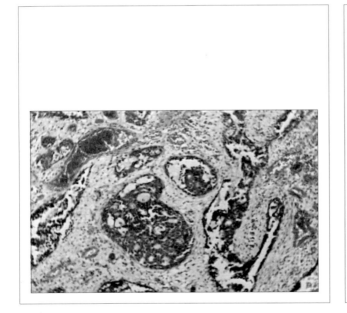

Figure 3 Adenocanthoma of the oesophagus showing the glandular differentiation part of the tumour (H & E)

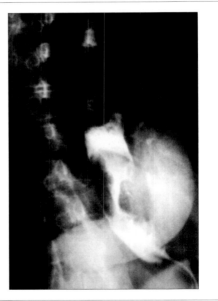

Figure 4 Radiograph of the oesophagus with a barium swallow in a female aged 52 years showing a large filling defect caused by a primary malignant melanoma

symptoms were inconstant, so that sometimes she felt well. Examination revealed no physical signs except tenderness high in the epigastrium.

Radiographs of the oesophagus with a barium swallow showed a neoplasm of the oesophagus involving approximately 7.5 cm in the upper limit and 12.5 cm in the lower limit, about 5 cm above the cardio-oesophageal orifice; there was a small amount of barium above this lesion (Figure 4). Oesophagoscopy showed a neoplasm causing rigidity of the oesophagus 25 cm from the incisor teeth, with marked dilatation of the oesophagus above it. Biopsy showed the histology of 'an anaplastic, very cellular carcinoma. There was no suggestion of glandular differentiation and it was thought to be of squamous origin'.

A partial oesophagogastrectomy with an oesophagogastric anastomosis was performed through a right thoracotomy following preliminary mobilization of the stomach through an upper abdominal incision. Palpation of the oesophagus revealed two tumours; there was no evidence of direct spread or intrathoracic metastases.

The patient made an uninterrupted recovery from the operation and was well for 5 months. She died 13 months later with disseminated malignant melanoma.

The surgical specimen consisted of the distal 12 cm of the oesophagus, the cardio-oesophageal junction and a ring of gastric tissue approximately 2 cm wide. In the upper part of the oesophagus was a non-pigmented polypoid tumour arising from a broad circular base 1.5 cm in diameter. Immediately below the tumour the oesophageal lumen was constricted; distal to this constriction and 1.5 cm from the tumour described there was a second large non-pigmented flat ulcerated tumour, which was neither polypoid nor pedunculated. It extended downwards for 5 cm almost to the cardio-oesophageal junction and occupied three-quarters of the oesophageal circumference, markedly narrowing the lumen. The mucosa

around the upper tumour and between the two tumours, and the narrow strip which remained uninvolved by the lower tumour, all appeared normal and showed no obvious pigmentation.

Blocks were taken from both tumours, from the oesophageal epithelium adjacent to both tumours, and from the intervening mucosa. Sections from each block were stained with haematoxylin and eosin. Masson–Fontana silver impregnation technique and Schmorl's technique with neutral red counterstain were used to identify melanin pigment. Hydrogen peroxide was used as a bleaching agent.

The upper polypoid tumour consisted of sheets of irregularly shaped pleomorphic cells arranged without pattern; tumour giant cells with multiple nuclei and cells in mitoses were moderately frequent. There was a clearly visible origin from the basal layer of oesophageal mucosa which showed conspicuous junctional change such as is seen in malignant melanomas and junctional naevi in the skin (Figure 5). The tumour was confined to the muscularis mucosae and had not invaded the submucosa or muscle coats; its clear origin from the epithelium proved it was not a metastasis. The majority of its cells were non-pigmented, but occasional tumour cells containing melanin pigment were present in it (Figure 6).

The lower tumour had a similar general histopathology appearance and tumour cells containing melanin pigment were present in it. It appeared to have originated in the submucosa and had ulcerated through the overlying epithelium, which was attenuated and did not show any junctional change, and had grown down into the muscle coats. The appearances suggested a secondary deposit from the upper tumour and this was borne out by the finding of submucosal islands of tumour between the two tumours.

The epithelium in the immediate vicinity of the upper pedunculated tumour also showed extensive

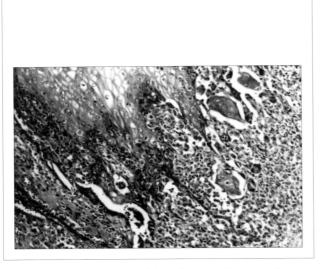

Figure 5 Histopathology of the primary malignant melanoma arising from the oesophageal epithelium showing junctional change (H & E)

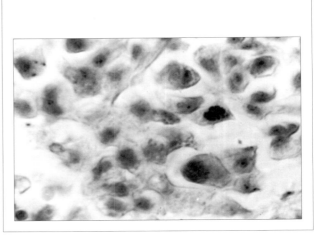

Figure 6 Histopathology of the primary malignant melanoma (Figure 5) showing melanin-containing tumour cells in the primary tumour (Masson–Fontana neutral red)

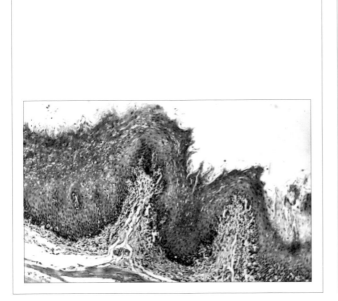

Figure 7 Histopathology of the primary malignant melanoma in the oesophagus (Figure 5) showing junctional changes in the epithelium adjacent to the primary tumour (H & E)

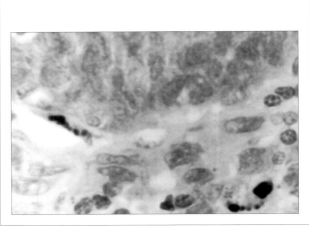

Figure 8 Histopathology of the primary malignant melanoma in the oesophagus (Figure 5) showing melanin-containing cells in the basal layers of the oesophageal epithelium and upper dermis (Masson–Fontana neutral red)

junctional changes (Figure 7). There were isolated small zones of junctional changes between the two tumours, but none below the upper limits of the lower tumour.

Melanin-containing cells resembling the melanoblasts and melanophores of the skin were present in these junctional zones (Figure 8) and there were very occasional similar cells in the epithelium of the upper and lower oesophagus which did not show junctional change.

The presence of melanoblasts in the epithelium of the oesophagus provides the basic reason for the occurrence of malignant melanoma in this organ. The tumour is large and fleshy, and pedunculated and polypoid or lobulated in appearance. It may be pigmented or non-pigmented; superficial ulceration is frequent and may cause considerable haemorrhage.

Raven and Dawson[4] point out that ideally the diagnosis should be based on the following criteria:

(1) The tumour should have the characteristic structure of a melanoma and contain pigment which is demonstrable as melanin by the appropriate staining techniques;

(2) It should arise from an area of junctional change in squamous epithelium[5];

(3) The adjacent epithelium should also show junctional changes with cells containing melanin pigment.

In practice the epithelium over the tumour is often ulcerated so that a direct origin from junctional epithelium may not be detected. Therefore if either criterion (2) or (3) is fulfilled the tumour can be regarded as a primary malignant melanoma.

REFERENCES

1. Kelly, A. B. (1919). Spasm at the entrance to the oesophagus. *J. Laryng.*, **34**, 285–9
2. Paterson, D. R. (1919). A clinical type of dysphagia. *J. Laryng.*, **34**, 289–91
3. Vinson, P. P. (1922). Hysterical dysphagia. *Minn. Med.*, **5**, 107
4. Raven, R. W. and Dawson, I. (1964). Malignant melanoma of the oesophagus. *Br. J. Surg.*, **51**, 551–5
5. Allen, A. C. and Spitz, S. (1953). Malignant melanoma: clinico-pathological analysis of criteria for diagnosis and prognosis. *Cancer*, **6**, 1–45

6

Tumours of the stomach

Carcinoma is the most frequent and important malignant tumour of the stomach, and it has a grave prognosis. The disease occurs more frequently in patients over the age of 50 years. There is evidence that gastric carcinoma incidence is raised in patients suffering from pernicious anaemia.

Attention is given here to two precancerous lesions in the stomach, namely the gastric adenomatous polyp and chronic gastric ulcer.

GASTRIC ADENOMATOUS POLYP

Adenomatous polyps develop in the stomach, colon and rectum and undoubtedly they can develop into carcinoma in these viscera. Gastric carcinoma is much more common than an adenomatous polyp in patients of the same age and sex. Multiple polyps may be present causing a higher risk of the development of a malignant tumour, and large polyps are more liable to become carcinomatous. Figure 1 shows the histopathology appearance of a benign adenomatous polyp of the stomach.

CHRONIC GASTRIC ULCER

There is no doubt that a carcinoma can develop in a chronic gastric ulcer, but this change seems to be somewhat rare. It is generally accepted that malignancy occurs in about 1% of cases, so that few carcinomas of the stomach originate in this way. The histopathology appearances of a chronic gastric ulcer undergoing malignant change are shown in Figures 2 and 3. Figure 4 shows the histopathology of a metastasis in the lung from a carcinoma which developed in a chronic gastric ulcer.

GASTRIC CARCINOMA

The basic type of carcinoma of the stomach is the mucin-secreting adenocarcinoma and there are several variations. There are two forms macroscopically, namely a malignant ulcer and a tumour which projects into the cavity of the stomach. A squamous cell carcinoma of the lower end of the oesophagus may extend into the proximal part of the stomach, and a carcinoma in the pancreas can invade the posterior gastric wall.

Histopathology
The adenocarcinoma shows various degrees of differentiation, from being well developed to an anaplastic tumour. There are variable amounts of mucin in the cells and stromal reaction may be minimal or gross.

Methods of spread
By direct extension The carcinoma spreads in the wall of the stomach, which may be penetrated to

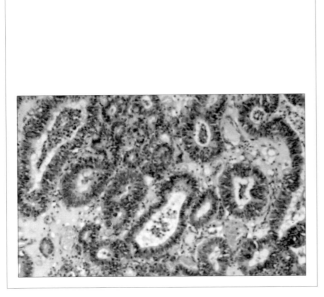

Figure 1 Histopathology appearance of a benign adenomatous polyp of the stomach

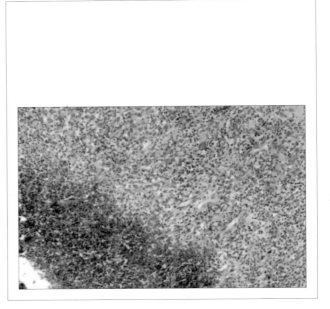

Figure 2 Histopathology appearance of the base of a chronic gastric ulcer

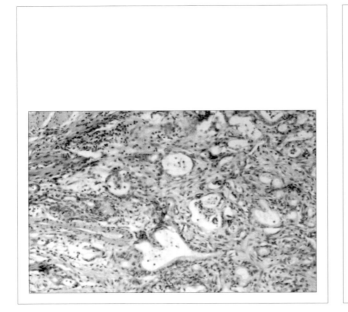

Figure 3 Histopathology appearance of a chronic gastric ulcer showing a carcinoma developing in the edge of the ulcer

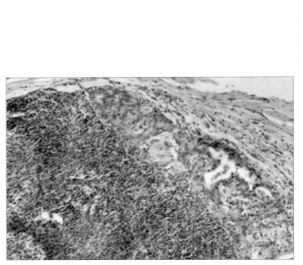

Figure 4 Histopathology appearance of a metastasis in the lung from a carcinoma which developed in a chronic gastric ulcer

involve the peritoneum, and invasion occurs into adjacent viscera including the pancreas and liver. The tumour may spread beyond the cardia into the lower end of the oesophagus but direct spread through the pylorus into the duodenum is very unusual.

By the lymphatics   Spread by the lymphatics to form metastases in the regional lymph nodes is both common and very serious. The disease soon spreads from the lymph nodes near the stomach to form metastases in the para-aortic and peripancreatic lymph nodes. Later the mediastinal and supraclavicular lymph nodes are involved.

By the bloodstream   Haematogenous metastases are seen chiefly in the liver and lungs, but widespread dissemination of the disease may occur.

By the peritoneum   Special mention is made of the spread of gastric carcinoma by the peritoneum whereby localized metastases are formed in the ovaries, especially of women in the younger age group. These tumours are known as Krukenberg tumours. Widespread small metastases develop in the pelvic peritoneum including the recto-uterine and rectovesical areas and malignant ascites may occur.

Carcinoma of the stomach in an advanced stage is seen less commonly than several decades ago because of earlier diagnosis in many patients, where gastroscopy has proved to be so valuable in allowing biopsy of the tumour and histopathological diagnosis. The early symptomatology of gastric carcinoma is often very mild. Included here are examples of advanced gastric carcinoma in patients who presented many years ago.

Case record   A male aged 65 years reported that for 6 months he had noticed that his upper abdomen was increasing in size and that he was anorexic. He noticed constipation but no vomiting and no cough. He felt that his food was held up in the lower gullet. He had experienced weight loss.

On examination the patient looked very ill, wasted and cachectic. No lymphadenopathy was present. Hypotension was noted. Examination showed the abdomen to be distended with ascites peritonei; there was marked hepatomegaly, the right lobe of the liver being larger than the left lobe, extending 5 cm below the umbilicus. The surface was nodular, especially in the middle of the right lobe where a large tumour was palpable.

X-ray examination with a barium meal showed a carcinoma involving the lower end of the oesophagus and the cardiac end of the stomach. The stomach was of the long J-shaped variety and the neoplasm seemed to extend about one-third of the way down along the lesser curvature. The upper end of the neoplasm lay a short distance above the hiatal canal and was causing a little obstruction with some hold-up of the barium, though most of the barium passed through the narrowed segment quite well. There seemed to be marked enlargement of the liver shadow and there was pleural thickening at the right base with a little parenchymal scarring consistent with previous inflammatory change. A gamma scan showed a large central defect in the liver with hepatomegaly.

The tumour was quite inoperable and a decision was made to give radiotherapy combined with chemotherapy. The patient's general nutritional state was first improved by intensive high-caloric feeding with vitamin supplementation and oral steroids. A course of quadruple cytotoxic chemotherapy was given followed by a course of radiotherapy to a dose of nearly 2000 R. A further course of chemotherapy followed.

The patient's general condition improved markedly with a weight gain of 5 kg in 2 weeks. There was shrinkage in the size of the liver with a decrease in ascitic fluid and peripheral oedema. The patient was eating well and was symptom-free. A repeat barium X-ray study showed substantial improvement, in that no more could be seen than a penetrating ulcer high up in the lesser curvature of the stomach and free flow of barium through the oesophagus. The patient then returned to his own country to continue chemotherapy including prednisolone and 5-fluoro-uracil (see Figures 5 and 6).

When a carcinoma of the stomach is operable, surgical treatment is carried out according to the position and size of the tumour in the stomach. When the tumour is localized to the distal segment, a partial gastrectomy is done; when a large tumour involves the body of the stomach, it is treated by a total gastrectomy and oesophagojejunal anastomosis. A carcinoma which involves the cardia and lower oesophagus is treated by a partial oesophagogastrectomy.

CARCINOMA IN A THORACIC STOMACH

The presence of either a portion or the whole of the stomach within the confines of the thorax is rare apart from an associated diaphragmatic hernia. The close embryonic relationship of the developing stomach and heart which is seen during the 4th week of embryonic life is soon estranged by the development of the diaphragm, when the stomach comes within the confines of the abdomen.

Percival Bailey enriched our knowledge of congenital anomalies by describing the viscera of a male patient who died aged 77 years. This patient had suffered no gastrointestinal or cardiac disturbances during his life, but anatomical dissection of his body after death revealed the stomach to be in the posterior mediastinum of the chest. Since this discovery, the condition of thoracic stomach associated with congenital shortening of the oesophagus has attracted the attention of clinicians and radiologists, who have published descriptions of the symptomatology and diagnosis.

It is a reasonable supposition that the same diseases which affect an intra-abdominal stomach will also affect an intrathoracic stomach, and therefore lesions such as benign and malignant ulcers and primary carcinoma should be encountered. A study of the literature concerning thoracic stomach failed to reveal a description of a case of carcinoma occurring in a thoracic stomach, so this pathological condition must be a rarity.

A patient with a primary carcinoma in a thoracic stomach came under the author's care and a study was made of the diagnosis and treatment[1].

The surgical treatment of this lesion was formulated by the author 50 years ago, when this operation had not previously been performed.

Case record A male aged 58 years was admitted to hospital complaining of vomiting half a pint of bright red blood 6 weeks previously. For several years he had experienced indigestion; he had had no pain or dysphagia and no recent weight loss. The patient's general condition was good; there were no cardiac or pulmonary abnormalities and his blood pressure was normal. There were no abdominal signs of any abnormality.

A radiogram with barium showed that the oesophagus was short, with a portion of the stomach within the chest, and an organic stricture was seen at the lower end of the oesophagus. Above the stricture there was slight dilatation, with reversed peristalsis (Figure 7). Oesophagoscopy showed a carcinoma at the lower end of the oesophagus 37 cm from the incisor teeth. Biopsy with histopathology showed fibrous tissue heavily infiltrated by poorly differentiated adenocarcinoma of a low columnar cell type. These features were more suggestive of a gastric carcinoma than of a carcinoma which originated in heterotopic gastric glands in the oesophageal mucosa.

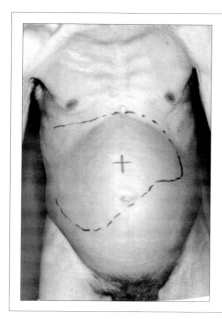

Figure 5 Clinical photograph of a male aged 65 years with an advanced carcinoma of the stomach causing metastases in the liver, with marked enlargement and ascites peritonei

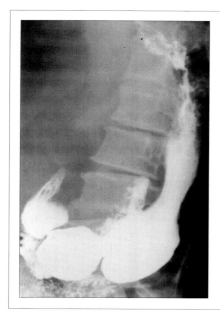

Figure 6 Radiological appearances in the same patient with a barium meal, showing a gastric carcinoma extending about one-third of the way down along the lesser curvature of the stomach and proximally involving the lower end of the oesophagus. There is marked hepatomegaly

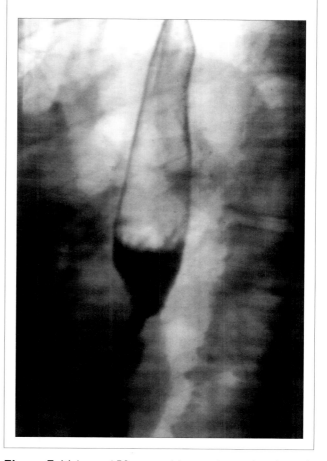

Figure 7 Male aged 58 years with a carcinoma in a thoracic stomach. Radiogram with barium showing a portion of the stomach in the chest and an organic stricture at the lower end of the oesophagus. Above the stricture there is slight dilatation of the oesophagus

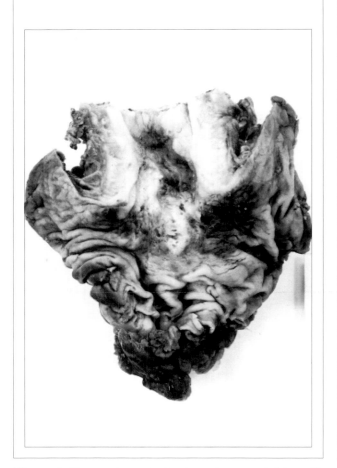

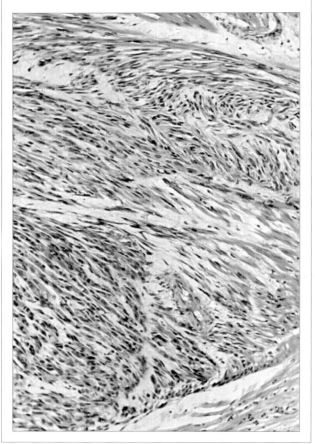

Figure 8 The carcinoma in the thoracic stomach (Figure 7) removed by left thoracotomy and thoraco-abdominal partial gastrectomy. The specimen shows the lower end of the oesophagus 2.5 cm long, opening into a saccular portion of the stomach 7.5 cm in diameter. In the stomach there is a carcinomatous ulcer 2.5 cm in diameter situated below and to the left of the cardiac orifice. There are no enlarged lymph nodes

Figure 9 Histopathology showing the typical appearance of leiomyosarcoma (H & E)

A preliminary anastomotic jejunostomy was performed for temporary feeding purposes. This was followed by a left thoracotomy and thoraco-abdominal partial gastrectomy with an oesophagogastric anastomosis. Figure 8 shows the surgical specimen.

Histopathology showed a fairly large well differentiated columnar cell adenocarcinoma of gastric origin infiltrating almost the whole thickness of the wall.

LEIOMYOSARCOMA

This is a rare malignant tumour of the stomach.

Case record   A male aged 52 years had been well until 8 months previously when he had developed increasing lassitude and anorexia. For the past 3 months he had had flatulence and upper abdominal discomfort, with no nausea or vomiting. During the last 2 months he had had attacks of constipation and diarrhoea and also melaena. A weight loss of 7 lb had been noted over 3 months. Recently the patient had noticed a mass in his upper abdomen.

On examination his general condition was good. A hard indefinite mass was palpable in the epigastrium. A radiogram with a barium meal showed a filling defect in the lower part of the stomach.

At operation, a very large vascular tumour was found in the middle third of the stomach. There was no evidence of metastases in the regional lymph nodes adjacent to the stomach, liver or peritoneal cavity. There was no free fluid in the abdomen. The large tumour was mobilized with difficulty and a partial gastrectomy was performed. Histopathology showed a leiomyosarcoma of the stomach (Figure 9).

Subsequently the patient returned to his own country following his recovery and he was quite well until 1 year and 3 months later when he began to lose weight. He later developed discomfort in his left thigh and 1 year and 10 months after the gastrectomy a radiogram of the pelvis showed destruction of the left innominate bone in the region of the left acetabulum due to an osteolytic metastasis. A course of radiotherapy was given in a dose of 3850 R which gave marked pain relief. The patient died in his country 2 years and 3 months after the gastrectomy was performed.

REFERENCE

1. Raven, R. W. (1941). Thoracico-abdominal gastrectomy for carcinoma of thoracic stomach. *Br. J. Surg.*, **29**, 39–46

7

Tumours of the colon, rectum and anus

Malignant tumours in the large bowel are common and several premalignant lesions are clearly recognized. Carcinoma of the colon is slightly more common in females than in males, but in the rectum the disease is more frequent in males. The age incidence is practically the same in both sexes.

TUMOURS OF THE COLON AND RECTUM

Premalignant lesions

Benign epithelial tumours

The close relationship between an adenoma and papilloma in the large bowel have been definitely established. Patients known to have a benign tumour and kept under observation for several years have developed a carcinoma and their symptoms of malignancy can be masked by the symptoms caused by a benign tumour. In addition, evidence of carcinoma can be found in a biopsy specimen of an adenoma or papilloma.

Familial polyposis of the colon and rectum

Familial polyposis is a hereditary disease which is rare. It is characterized by the development of large numbers of adenomas, which are sessile and polypoid, throughout the colon and rectum. There is excessive proliferation of the glandular component of the intestinal mucous membrane which leads to the formation of these benign tumours. This disease occurs with equal frequency in males and in females and either partner can transmit it to children. A number of these patients will develop a carcinoma in the colon or rectum which is indicated by an increase in size and later ulceration of the affected polyp. An illustration is shown in Figure 1 of a female aged 26 years with familial polyposis who developed a carcinoma of the ascending colon.

Ulcerative colitis

Carcinoma may develop in patients with severe ulcerative colitis affecting the whole colon and rectum after this disease has been present for many years and persists. An unsuspected carcinoma may be discovered in the colon when total colectomy has been performed for chronic ulcerative colitis; this complication will become less common now that this radical operation is performed more frequently in the earlier phase of this disease.

Malignant tumours of the colon

Carcinoma is the common malignant tumour of the colon; sarcoma is rare and usually it is a lymphoid or reticulum variety although leiomyosarcoma may occur. Carcinoma is more common in the pelvic colon than in the other parts, where the caecum and adjacent ascending colon preponderate over the transverse and descending sectors. Multiple carcinomas may be present so that a careful examination must be made of the whole colon when surgical treatment is performed.

These tumours in the colon resemble those in the rectum although their relative frequency is different.

Proliferative carcinoma

This is a bulky tumour which projects into the lumen of the bowel and usually does not penetrate deeply through the muscle of the bowel wall and the adjacent tissue. The tumour remains localized for some time as it is slow to form metastases. Histopathology generally shows a well differentiated adenocarcinoma.

Ulcerative carcinoma

This variety of carcinoma is the common variety in the rectum but it does occur in the colon second in frequency to the proliferative type of tumour. The malignant ulcer spreads in the wall of the bowel, which may be encircled, and it has the characteristic features with a raised, hard, everted edge. The tumour penetrates deeply into and through the bowel wall into adjacent tissue and forms metastases relatively early.

Scirrhous carcinoma

This variety of tumour contains much fibrous tissue and it spreads completely around the bowel, causing a hard complete stricture with severe narrowing of the lumen. Thus complete intestinal obstruction can occur.

Methods of spread

By direct extension   The Dukes' classification records the extent of local spread of the carcinoma in correlation with lymphatic and venous spread. This classification is usually applied to the stage of rectal carcinoma but it is also applicable to colonic carcinoma. According to the classification, in the first stage the carcinoma is limited to the bowel – 'A' case. In the second stage the tumour has spread by direct extension through the bowel wall into adjacent structures but there are no lymph node metastases – 'B' case. In the third case, lymph node metastases are present; when only the regional lymph nodes are involved it is termed a 'C' case, but if lymph nodes extend to the ligation of the blood vessels it is a 'C2' case.

In carcinoma of the colon there are more cases in the 'A' group than in rectal carcinoma.

By the lymphatics   Usually carcinoma metastases are formed in the regional lymph nodes when the tumour has spread through the muscle coat of the wall of the bowel into the peritoneum or other adjacent tissues. Some carcinomas are anaplastic with high metastatic potential and form lymph node metastases early; in such cases the prognosis is unfavourable following surgical treatment.

Blood-borne metastases   There is evidence of carcinoma spread in the veins in some specimens removed surgically, where a solid core of tumour is found in an adjacent vein resembling local spread of the carcinoma. Otherwise carcinoma cells can pass into the venous system and metastases in the liver, lungs and other viscera are not infrequent from colonic and rectal carcinoma.

Carcinoma of the colon may be associated with other colonic diseases such as diverticular disease.

Case record   A female aged 52 years presented with the following history. Until 9 months earlier her bowel habit had been regular and then she had become constipated and this problem had become worse. On one occasion she had passed bright red blood. She had experienced pain at times in the right lower abdomen. At age 49 years she had undergone a perineorrhaphy.

Rectal examination revealed a rectocele with poor tone of the anorectal sphincters, which caused rectal incontinence. Radiological examination showed moderate diverticulitis of the pelvic colon and lower part

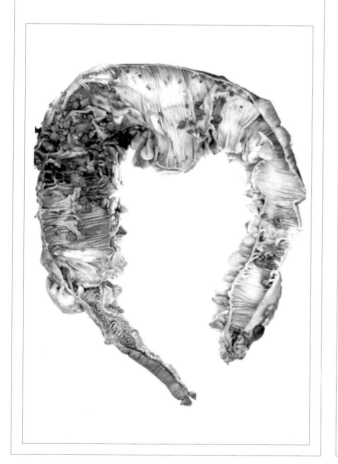

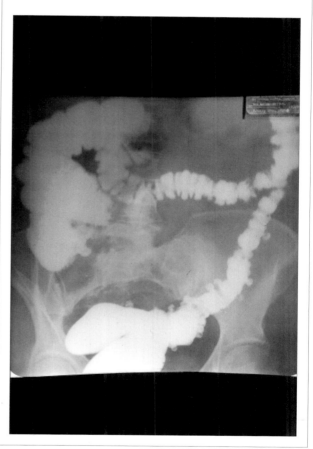

Figure 1 Female with polyposis of the colon who developed a carcinoma in the ascending colon aged 26 years. A total colectomy was performed as shown in the illustration. She developed recurrent carcinoma 1 year later

Figure 2 Radiogram with a barium enema of a female aged 52 years with a carcinoma in the sigmoid colon associated with diverticulosis of the descending colon. A perineal repair of the rectocele was performed and the diverticulitis was treated medically.

The patient was referred again 3 years later. She had had complete rectal continence since the reconstruction operation to her anorectal sphincters. She had developed constipation one year earlier with increasing pain in the left lower quadrant of the abdomen, accompanied by fever. On abdominal examination a firm tender swelling in the left iliac fossa was found. Rectal examination showed good sphincteric tone.

The patient's diverticulitis had progressed considerably (Figure 2) so that surgical treatment was indicated; at the same operation a colonic carcinoma was to be considered.

An exploratory laparotomy was performed. This confirmed the diverticulitis and a carcinoma of the sigmoid colon associated with diverticulitis was found. A left hemicolectomy was performed. The patient made a good recovery from the operation.

The surgical specimen consisted of 62 cm of the colon. In the middle of the specimen and completely encircling the bowel there was a raised papilliferous tumour extending along the bowel for a distance of 4 cm. On sectioning, the tumour appeared to be infiltrating the muscle coats but had not spread into the surrounding pericolic fat. No other polypoid lesions were seen in the colon. Above and below the tumour there were numerous diverticula with wide necks. The muscle coats were greatly thickened, and the wall of the colon was thrown into numerous small folds. No mucosal ulceration other than in the tumour area could be seen.

Histopathology showed a well differentiated adenocarcinoma. It had just penetrated the muscle coats and there was very little invasion of the pericolic fat. The blood vessels appeared free of growth. The

ten lymph nodes sectioned showed a well marked follicular hyperplasia, but were all free of growth. One section showed several diverticula, thickening of the muscle coats, and prominent mucosal folds. No inflammatory reaction was seen. A diagnosis of carcinoma of the colon with diverticulosis was made.

Case record A male aged 68 years was seen with griping pain in the lower half of the abdomen for 10 weeks. More recently his bowels had been a little loose; there had been no blood in the stools. His father died aged 47 of lymphoma and his mother had died aged 67 of cancer of the rectum.

Examination showed a little tenderness in the left iliac fossa; no rectal abnormality was found. Radiograms of the colon with a barium enema were very suggestive of a neoplasm of the pelvic colon about 10 cm above the pelvirectal junction. There was some obstruction in the pelvic colon and large diverticula were present in the colon.

A partial colectomy for carcinoma in the pelvic colon associated with diverticulosis (Figure 3) was performed. The patient made a good recovery from the operation.

Figure 4 shows another example of a carcinoma of the colon, removed by partial colectomy in an 86-year-old woman.

A carcinoma of the hepatic flexure of the colon may invade the adjacent right lobe of the liver by direct extension.

Case record A male aged 38 years gave this history. One year earlier when in India he had developed pain in the right lower abdomen which was sharp and accompanied by diarrhoea. This attack had subsided, but several weeks later the diarrhoea had recurred with four stools daily. Pain in the right lower abdomen had become continuous 7 months before consultation; anorexia had developed and he had become

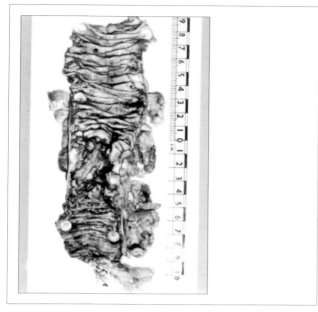

Figure 3 Male aged 68 years with a carcinoma of the pelvic colon associated with diverticulosis. The specimen shows the distal colon with the carcinoma and the large diverticula

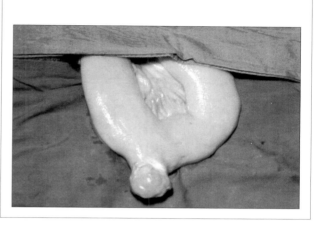

Figure 4 Female aged 86 years with a carcinoma of the colon treated by partial colectomy. The operation specimen shows a carcinoma with an unusual tongue-like projection of the tumour through the bowel wall

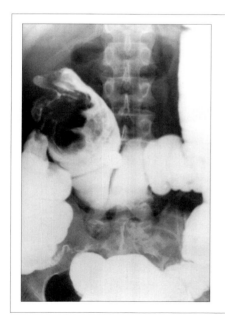

Figure 5 The surgical specimen of the massive carcinoma of the hepatic flexure of the colon invading the right lobe of the liver, treated by a right hemicolectomy and partial hepatectomy (right lobe)

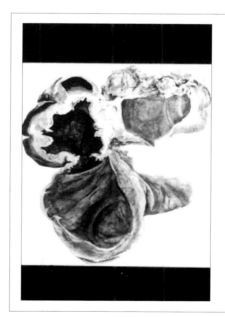

Figure 6 Male aged 38 years with a large carcinoma of the hepatic flexure of the colon invading the right lobe of the liver showing the appearances in a radiogram with a barium enema

constipated and had gradually lost strength. Three months earlier he had returned to Britain and had been admitted to another hospital. A hard mass had been noted in the right hypochondrium, blood was present in the stools and *Entamoeba histolytica* was demonstrated. A radiogram with a barium enema at that time showed a large filling defect in the transverse colon. A course of emetine was given to exclude an amoeboma, without any effect. Following a blood transfusion an exploratory laparotomy was performed and the mass appeared to be a large scirrhous carcinoma of the transverse colon just medial to the hepatic flexure and invading the gall bladder and liver to which it was densely adherent; no metastases were found. The carcinoma was considered inoperable so an ileotransverse colostomy was performed. The patient made a good recovery, the abdominal pain subsided, stools returned to normal and his appetite improved.

Later his condition deteriorated, with the development of severe secondary anaemia and in spite of three blood transfusions of 1 pint (568 ml) each, the red blood corpuscles fell to $2.4 \times 10^6/mm^3$ and the haematocrit to 35%. Severe pain developed in the tumour area.

On examination the patient looked ill and had lost much weight. There was a large mass in the right half of the abdomen extending from the right hypochondrium to the upper limit of the right iliac fossa, somewhat fixed and extremely tender. Sigmoidoscopy was negative and a bowel smear showed no cysts or amoebae. There was marked secondary anaemia, red blood corpuscles numbered $1.9 \times 10^6/mm^3$ and the haematocrit was 28%. A radiogram with a barium enema showed a large irregular filling defect at the hepatic flexure of the colon extending 5 cm into the transverse colon and 10 cm into the caecum. This had the appearance of a carcinoma (Figure 5).

The patient was given three blood transfusions of 3 pints (1.7 l), 1.5 pints (0.85 l) and 5 pints (2.84 l).

The last massive transfusion was given because of a rapid deterioration in his general condition, probably due to haemorrhage from the colonic carcinoma. It was decided – and the patient and his wife wished it – to perform an exploratory laparotomy to determine whether the tumour could be removed. This operation was performed and the large carcinoma involving the hepatic flexure of the colon and the right lobe of the liver was found. No metastases were in the rest of the liver or elsewhere in the abdomen and the ileotransverse colostomy was perfectly satisfactory. A right partial hepatectomy combined with a right hemicolectomy was performed. The patient made a good recovery (Figure 6).

Histopathology showed a highly cellular adenocarcinoma[1].

TUMOURS OF THE RECTUM

Carcinoma
Tumours, both benign and malignant, develop quite frequently in the rectum. There are several well known precancerous lesions in the rectum and reference has been made to benign epithelial tumours, familial polyposis and severe ulcerative colitis of longstanding, where carcinoma may supervene later.

Carcinoma is the most frequent tumour in the rectum. Sarcomas are rare and they form bulky tumours which project into the rectal lumen and are softer in consistency. Lymphoma occurs and may be multiple. Many features of rectal carcinoma resemble those already described for colonic carcinoma.

Spread of carcinoma of the rectum
By direct extension   This method of spread is more dangerous than in colonic carcinoma because of the close proximity of the rectum to other important pelvic viscera which are often invaded. Thus infiltration of the prostate, seminal vesicles and base of the bladder occurs when the carcinoma is situated in the

lower two-thirds of the rectum, and this causes problems in surgical treatment.

In females, a carcinoma in the lower two-thirds of the rectum in the anterior wall may become attached to the rectovaginal septum and penetrate into the vagina, causing a malignant rectovaginal fistula. Carcinoma in the upper third of the rectum at the peritoneal reflection becomes adherent to the cervix and corpus uteri, and malignant invasion occurs which necessitates a more radical pelvic operation.

The carcinoma in the rectum ulcerates into the rectouterine pouch or rectovesical pouch. If this occurs a loop of small intestine may become adherent to the tumour.

By the lymphatics Metastases are found frequently in the regional lymph nodes, especially in the anaplastic highly malignant carcinoma. The pararectal nodes close to the tumour are affected first, followed by the superior haemorrhoidal group. Further upward lymphatic spread can occur as high as the ligation of the inferior mesenteric blood vessels in the operation of abdominoperineal excision of the rectum. A carcinoma in the lower part of the rectum and anal canal may form metastases in the inguinal lymph nodes.

By the blood vessels Blood-borne metastases are more likely to form from the anaplastic highly malignant carcinomas and especially when the tumour has progressed through the rectal wall into the region of the veins. Metastases form in the liver and lungs and also in other viscera.

Figures 7–12 are examples of carcinoma of the rectum from several patients.

Case record A female aged 57 years was referred with an advanced carcinoma of the rectum causing sciatica. She had been constipated for 8 weeks with rectal pain and blood in her stools. Abdominal examination showed distension of the pelvic colon with faeces. Rectal examination revealed a hard ulcerating carcinoma in the rectum, 8 cm from the anal verge, which was infiltrating the posterior vaginal fornix. An abdominoperineal excision of the rectum combined with a Wertheim's hysterectomy was performed. The patient made a good recovery from the operation.

Figure 13 shows the operation specimen. In the rectum with its lower margin 8 cm from the recto-anal junction there was a deep carcinomatous ulcer 5.5 cm in its widest diameter with a fungating margin which extended through all coats and for a distance of about 2.5 cm into the surrounding connective tissues posteriorly. Anteriorly it was bound to the uterus at the level of the cervix uteri by secondary growth. The uterus was small with a calcified pedunculated serosal fibroid. The ovaries and fallopian tubes were normal.

Histopathology showed a very anaplastic carcinoma composed of large pleomorphic cells invading all coats of the bowel and extending massively into the surrounding tissues.

Figure 14 is an example of rectal carcinoma invading the vagina, causing a malignant rectovaginal fistula.

Advanced carcinomas of the rectum with direct extension into the uterus and vagina in addition to invasion of other viscera and tissues in the pelvis will become increasingly uncommon in the future due to routine medical check-ups, and to early diagnosis of carcinoma because of patient awareness to seek medical advice for suspicious symptoms. The indication for the major operation of combined abdominoperineal excision of the rectum and Wertheim's hysterectomy will therefore decrease.

Argentaffinoma (carcinoid) tumours of the rectum

Patients with an argentaffinoma of the rectum can be divided into three main groups[2].

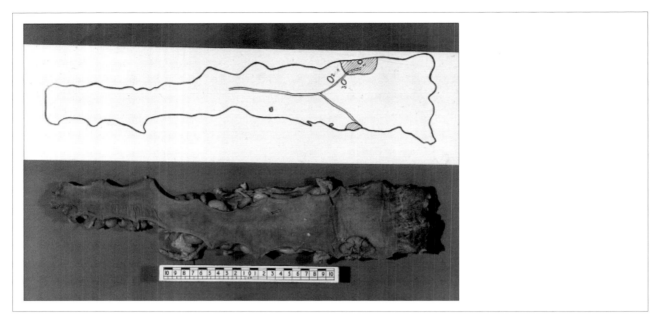

Figure 7 Specimen of rectum showing a carcinoma and polyps

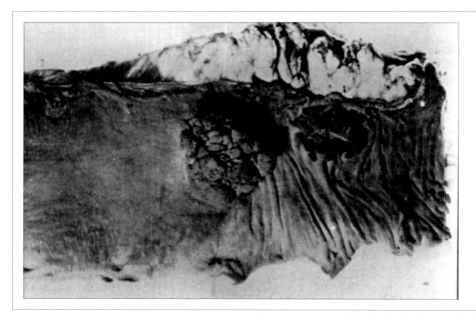

Figure 8 Specimen of rectum showing a carcinoma and a papilloma

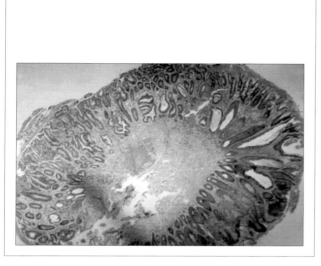

Figure 9 Histopathology of carcinoma *in situ* of the rectum under low power magnification (H & E)

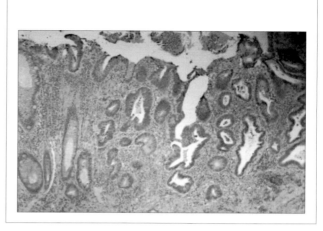

Figure 10 The same tumour under high power magnification (H & E). The sections show marked irregularity in the size and shape of the epithelial cells. There are irregular foci of carcinoma cells and considerable intercellular oedema is present

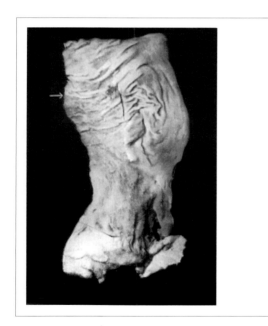

Figure 11 Specimen showing a very early carcinoma of the rectum diagnosed by sigmoidoscopy and biopsy. A perineal excision of the rectum was performed

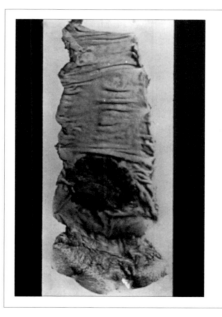

Figure 12 Specimen showing a carcinoma of the rectum of the sessile papilliferous variety

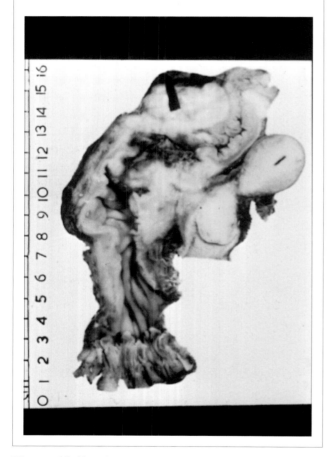

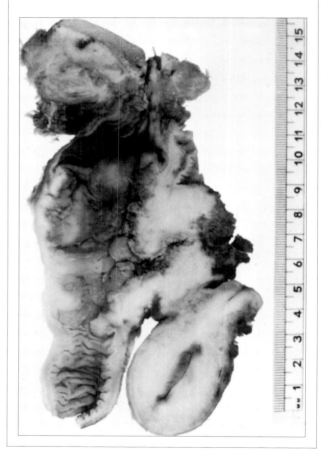

Figure 13 Female aged 57 years with an advanced carcinoma of the rectum infiltrating the corpus and cervix uteri through the posterior vaginal fornix. Operation specimen from an abdominoperineal excision of the rectum combined with a Wertheim's hysterectomy

Figure 14 Female with an advanced carcinoma in the lower third of the rectum invading the vagina and causing a malignant rectovaginal fistula. Specimen following an abdominoperineal excision of the rectum combined with a Wertheim's hysterectomy

Asymptomatic cases The argentaffinoma is discovered in the rectum as the result of an examination for some other condition such as a fissure or haemorrhoids. It may also be found in the operation specimen of a rectum which was removed for a carcinoma.

Metastatic cases The patient may present with symptoms due to metastases of argentaffinoma in other viscera, especially the liver, the primary tumour in the rectum being silent. The chief symptoms in this group include anorexia, nausea, increasing fatigue and weight loss. There may be the important flushing of the skin.

Cases with rectal symptoms The chief symptoms of patients in this group are rectal bleeding, either bright red or dark red in colour; a change in bowel habit, with constipation of increasing severity, or diarrhoea; and tenesmus. The argentaffinoma may be single and usually arises in the anterior wall of the rectum; it may be completely submucosal, but in other cases there is a partial covering of mucous membrane. It is freely mobile unless infiltrative properties have developed. The type of tumour is variable; thus a nodule, polyp, plaque or annular constriction may be felt. Its consistency is rubbery or firm and sometimes there is infiltration of surrounding tissues. The size may equal that of any malignant rectal tumour. On inspection the colour of the tumour varies from white or yellow to red-brown. Multiple argentaffinomas may occur.

The differential diagnosis depends upon the type of argentaffinoma which is present. When pedunculated, it must be distinguished from an adenomatous polyp; if it is submucous, from benign connective tissue tumours and inflammatory swellings; and when the argentaffinoma is infiltrative it must be distinguished from a carcinoma and lymphogranuloma inguinale.

Case record A female aged 60 years complained of continuous pain in the rectum and tenesmus. She had been constipated for many years. She had no rectal bleeding or diarrhoea. A polyp arising in the right lateral wall 3 cm from the anal verge, firm in consistency, was found. Large internal haemorrhoids were also present. Sigmoidoscopy showed no other abnormality up to 20 cm from the anal verge. A haemorrhoidectomy and excision of the polyp was performed. Histopathology showed the structure of the polyp to be that of an argentaffinoma.

One year and 6 months later the patient was well; there was no recurrent or metastatic argentaffinoma.

An argentaffinoma must be regarded as a malignant tumour, for in some patients widespread metastases occur. The tumour progresses slowly and the malignant potential is less than that of adenocarcinoma. As the tumour enlarges, its cells will eventually transgress their barriers and infiltrate adjacent tissues and metastasize.

When an argentaffinoma has been excised in the belief that it was an adenomatous polyp, subsequent histopathology proving the diagnosis, the patient is kept under observation to detect any recurrence. When a small, non-infiltrating argentaffinoma is found and confirmed by histopathology, a wide local excision is performed and the patient kept under observation. A radical operation when a large argentaffinoma with infiltrating properties is present, or when there is an annular constricting argentaffinoma. If a recurrent argentaffinoma develops, a radical operation should be performed.

TUMOURS OF THE ANUS AND ANAL CANAL

Carcinoma is the usual malignant tumour that occurs in the anal canal and anus and the disease here is much less frequent than carcinoma of the rectum. The anal canal may be affected by the direct spread of carcinoma in the lower third of the rectum.

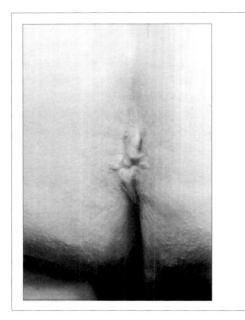

Figure 15 Female aged 68 years with a recurrent squamous cell carcinoma of the anal verge which was excised with a margin of normal tissue

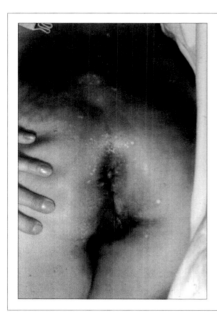

Figure 16 Female aged 59 years with an extensive adenocarcinoma of the lower third of the rectum extending into the anal canal, posterior vaginal wall, perirectal tissues and left ischiorectal fossa. Inflammatory changes are shown

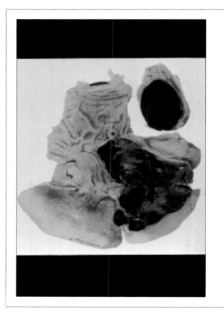

Figure 17 Specimen of a rectum, anal canal and anus excised because of a malignant melanoma of the anus and anal canal invading the rectum. A large black metastasis is present in the lymph node

The histology of the anal canal changes as we proceed from the anorectal junction to the anal orifice. Thus, in the upper part there is columnar epithelium with simple tubular glands which gradually merges into stratified columnar and polygonal epithelium. The lower half of the anal canal is lined first by modified squamous stratified epithelium with a few papillae and this merges at the anal verge into the squamous epithelium of skin.

The majority of malignant tumours in the upper half of the anal canal are basal cell carcinomas, while most of the tumours in the lower half are squamous cell carcinomas. Tumours with mixed histopathology also occur, which are partly adenocarcinoma and partly squamous carcinoma. A basal cell carcinoma may occur in the skin of the anal verge with the characteristic features of this tumour in the skin of other parts of the body.

Carcinoma of the anal canal spreads locally by direct extension into the surrounding muscles. These tumours also metastasize to the regional lymph nodes. Thus, upward spread occurs into the haemorrhoidal group of lymph nodes, and the tumours spread by the lymphatic vessels laterally and downwards to cause metastases in the inguinal group of lymph nodes.

Case record A female aged 68 years had noticed accidentally by touch a small pointed projection about the lower edge of the anus whilst applying cream, 8 days previously. This projection had disappeared within 24 h. Her past history was important because 8 months previously an excision of a 'condyloma' of the anal verge had been performed at another hospital at the same site as the present swelling, but it had been more extensive. Histopathology showed a well differentiated squamous cell carcinoma.

On examination of the anus an ulcer was found at the right anterior aspect of the anal verge, 1 cm in diameter, and mobile on the underlying muscle sphincter (Figure 15). The rest of the anal canal and rectum were normal. Biopsy and histopathology showed a superficially infiltrating poorly keratinizing squamous cell carcinoma. The inguinal lymph nodes were not enlarged.

A wide local excision of the ulcerating carcinoma was performed. Histopathology sections showed a small central localized area of superficially infiltrating well differentiated squamous cell carcinoma. Excision was complete.

The patient made a good recovery and the wound gradually healed.

The anal canal can be involved by a carcinoma extending into it from the rectum.

Case record A female aged 59 years had experienced central abdominal pain, colicky in nature, 4 months earlier. 1 week earlier she had noticed a small lump in the upper medial left buttock. Examination showed a small nodular tumour protruding through the anal orifice and invading the left ischiorectal fossa where the skin was red and inflammatory changes present. Rectal examination was too painful and required an anaesthetic. A fungating tumour was found in the lower third of the rectum extending down the anal canal, which was surrounded by tumour; this had spread through the posterior vaginal wall and into the left ischiorectal fossa causing an abscess (Figure 16). Biopsy and histopathology showed a moderately differentiated adenocarcinoma consistent with an origin in the rectum.

The operation performed consisted of:

(1) A left inguinal colostomy and antibiotic therapy with marked improvement in the patient's general condition and perineal inflammation;

(2) A laparotomy for strangulated loops of small intestine prolapsed between the colostomy and

left lateral abdominal wall; the loops were easily reduced and the lateral space occluded; and

(3) An abdominoperineal excision of the rectum combined with the excision of the total posterior vaginal wall, cervix and corpus uteri, and clearance of the left ischiorectal fossa and right side of the pelvis. The pelvic floor was reconstructed. The patient made a good recovery from this operation.

Histopathology showed a well differentiated adenocarcinoma of the rectum, penetrating the whole thickness of the rectal and vaginal walls, with wide infiltration of perirectal tissues on both lateral aspects. There were no lymph node metastases. The tumour was of low grade malignancy. The margin of tumour clearance was wide in the sections examined.

Malignant melanoma of the anorectum

The anorectal region is the commonest site in the alimentary tract to be affected by primary malignant melanoma, but even here the number of cases reported in the literature is not large. Raven[3] noted that up to that time only 100 cases had been reported in the literature; W. E. Miles was quoted in his statement that he had seen only three cases in more than 1500 cases of carcinoma of the rectum. Raven also reported that during the previous 15 years he had found the case records of only three patients with this disease admitted to the Royal Cancer Hospital[3]. The following are details of those patients.

The first case was a male aged 59 years who had experienced increasing constipation for 9 months and a sense of rectal obstruction. Morning diarrhoea was present and 'rectal prolapse' occurred, diagnosed elsewhere as 'piles'. Stools were ribbon-like; there was no blood or mucus. Examination showed abdominal distension in the region of the caecum. A tumour was present in the posterior wall of the anal canal filling the lumen and extending down to the level of the white line. Hard, shotty lymph nodes were

palpable in the left groin. An exploratory laparotomy revealed multiple nodules in the small intestine, a small hard nodule in the vault of the urinary bladder and two large masses in the rectovesical pouch. The anal tumour was excised locally and diathermy applied to the base. Histopathology showed the tumour to be a malignant melanoma; pigment formation was minimal. The tumour was composed mainly of cells of epithelial type, but in one part showed a tendency to a spindle form. Small strands of necrotic squamous epithelium, a few tubular mucus-secreting glands and occasional unstriped muscle fibres were the only traces of normal structure in the specimen.

The second case was a male aged 39 years who had experienced severe bleeding and discharge from the rectum and faecal incontinence. A lump at the anus was noticed. Examination showed that the abdomen was distended and a tumour, 4 × 3 cm, purplish and firm in consistency, protruded from the anus. This tumour extended high up the anal canal and induration was present in the ischiorectal fossae. There were firm lymph nodes in both groins. At exploratory laparotomy, a large tumour was found involving the rectum with extension to the right side of the pelvis. The liver was normal. Excision of the rectum was not possible; a left inguinal colostomy was instituted. The protruding tumour at the anus was excised by diathermy 19 days later.

Histopathology showed the tumour to be a malignant melanoma. It was partially covered by squamous epithelium which was partly hyperplastic, partly atrophic and partly ulcerated. The malignant parenchyme showed considerable heterogeneity and many parts were completely achromic. Other parts showed melanin pigmentation in both melanoblasts and chromatophores. The component cells were sometimes fusiform or polyhedral, but there were many circumscribed lobulated masses of cells of large spherical form bearing a striking resemblance to neuro-epithelial end-organs. Mitotic figures and examples of nuclear hyperchromia, reduplication and syncytium formation were abundant and the tumour was extremely malignant.

The third case was a male aged 62 years who had experienced pain on sitting down for 3 months, and rectal bleeding for 6 weeks. A colostomy had been performed elsewhere 6 weeks earlier. Examination showed a purplish-brown tumour occupying the anus, extending outward to the buttock and upward along the full length of the anal canal. The rectal mucosa beyond the tumour appeared normal. The tumour was firm in consistency and did not bleed when touched. A perineal excision of the rectum was performed. After 19 days the patient underwent excision of the left inguinal lymph nodes. Histopathology showed an actively growing, extensively pigmented malignant melanoma. There was massive infiltration of the regional lymph nodes by malignant melanoma, but the highest lymph node removed showed no invasion. The left inguinal lymph nodes showed massive invasion by malignant melanoma.

Site of origin

A malignant melanoma usually arises in the anal canal or at the anal verge. It is very exceptional for the tumour to commence in the rectum but this may be involved by direct extension from the anal canal. The posterior wall of the anal canal is more often involved than the others, followed by the lateral walls; the anterior wall is the most infrequent site.

The tumour usually forms a single mass, but a second smaller tumour is sometimes present separated by apparently normal tissue. There may be a small anal tumour with a large one in the rectal ampulla, or the primary tumour may be surrounded by a number of small satellites. The size of a malignant melanoma in this region varies from a miliary nodule to a large tumour, with many intermediate varieties.

Types of tumour

There are two main types, sessile and pedunculated. It is a special feature of the malignant melanoma in this region to become pedunculated, which explains the frequency with which it prolapses through the anal orifice. The tumour base is frequently mobile over the deeper layers of the anal canal. The tumour is usually lobulated and areas of superficial ulceration may be present. It is frequently black due to melanin; an amelanotic type may be present. The consistency is firm and elastic; sometimes it feels semifluctuant.

Spread of the tumour

Direct extension Malignant melanoma commencing in the anal canal has a marked tendency to spread upwards into the rectum along the submucous tissues. It also spreads outwards into the cellular tissues surrounding the anus and rectum, but this appears to be resisted by the fascia propria of the rectum. Unlike adenocarcinoma, malignant melanoma does not usually invade adjacent structures such as the urinary bladder, vagina or sacrum. Tumour nodules may be found in the ischiorectal fossa, or in the cellular tissues in the hollow of the sacrum.

Lymphatic spread The inguinal lymph nodes are frequently involved by metastases. If only one lateral wall of the anal canal is affected the lymph nodes on that particular side may be involved, the others being normal. It is necessary to distinguish between chromatophores and actual malignant melanoma cells in the lymph nodes. When the rectum is involved its lymph nodes are invaded as in adenocarcinoma. Usually lymph node metastases are black, although the primary tumour may be amelanotic. Involvement of the lymphatic system may be more generalized to include the thoracic duct, mesenteric, mediastinal and submaxillary groups of lymph nodes.

Haematogenous spread Invasion of the blood vessels by the tumour causes widespread metastases, but dissemination may be delayed for a considerable time. The liver is involved most frequently, causing enlargement and nodularity. These nodules may be black or amelanotic. The peritoneum may be studded with neoplastic nodules and metastases may be present in the small intestines, greater omentum and appendices epiploica. The lungs and pleura are involved frequently. The subcutaneous tissues, kidney, brain and meninges, pancreas, spleen and thyroid gland may be affected.

Symptomatology

A common symptom is the presence of a mass protruding from the anal orifice which may be mistaken for a prolapsed thrombosed internal haemorrhoid. Bleeding and discharge are frequent. There may be bowel action irregularity with frequency of defaecation and tenesmus. The protruding tumour is dark brown or black, or a nodular pedunculated mass can be felt in the anal canal and a blackish discharge is noted on the examining finger. The regional lymph nodes may be enlarged and tender. In advanced cases a large mass of lymph nodes is present and ulceration with suppuration may occur.

The primary tumour must be distinguished from a prolapsed ulcerated internal haemorrhoid and when doubt exists biopsy is done and histopathology determined.

Treatment

An exploratory laparotomy is carried out to determine tumour extensions and operability. When conditions are favourable, an abdominoperineal excision of the rectum and anus should be performed. After 3 or 4 weeks a bilateral block dissection of lymph nodes in both groins is carried out. On the whole, malignant melanoma is not radiosensitive, so that whenever possible radical surgical excision is performed. Figure 17 shows a specimen obtained from such a procedure.

REFERENCES

1. Raven, R. W. (1947). Partial hepatectomy and right hemi-colectomy for carcinoma of the hepatic flexure. *Br. Med. J.,* **2**, 249–50
2. Raven, R. W. (1950). Carcinoid tumours of the rectum. *Proc. Roy. Soc. Med.,* **43**, 675–7
3. Raven, R. W. (1948). Ano-rectal malignant melanoma. *Proc. Roy. Soc. Med.,* **41**, 469–74

8

Tumours of the breast

Tumours in the breast, both benign and malignant varieties, are common in females but rare in males. Clinical and laboratory research concerning these tumours have clarified problems of breast pathology and also of tumour pathology as a whole. Considerable ongoing research continues throughout the world for there are many important questions which require an answer. For example, we need a clear understanding of hormonal control mechanisms to be applied in the hormonal treatment of breast carcinoma.

BENIGN TUMOURS OF THE FEMALE BREAST

Fibroadenoma
Small fibroadenomas occur in association with adenosis and cystic hyperplasia and usually regress with increasing fibrosis of the breast tissues. A larger fibroadenoma may develop in young women and is usually excised with its fibrous capsule. The stroma is the most active component in these tumours and very rarely a sarcoma supervenes.

Papilloma
A small solitary papilloma may occur in the main duct of the breast near the nipple and cause a blood-stained discharge (Figures 1 and 2). Multiple small papillomas develop in small ducts deeper in the breast

in association with cystic hyperplasia (Figure 3). A breast papilloma may become malignant forming an intraduct carcinoma with infiltrative potential (Figures 4 and 5). A duct papilloma causing nipple bleeding is treated by a small segmental resection of the breast.

MALIGNANT TUMOURS IN THE FEMALE BREAST

Carcinoma
Carcinoma of the breast is the commonest malignant tumour in women in the Western world. The disease usually occurs in the age group 40–60 years, but both younger and older women may be affected.

Site of the carcinoma
The upper outer quadrant of the breast is the commonest site for the tumour to develop, followed by the central area and upper inner quadrant. The lower half of the breast is affected much less commonly; sometimes the carcinoma causes diffuse breast enlargement. The opposite breast may be affected by spread of tumour from a breast, or a second primary carcinoma may develop there later, so that this breast must continue under observation.

Spread of the disease
By direct extension　Carcinoma is considered to have a multicentric origin in the breast tissue and these foci

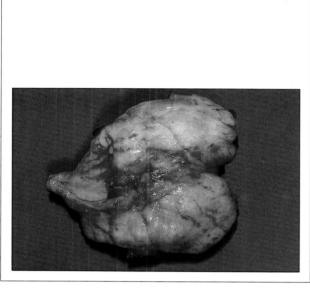

Figure 1 Specimen of a large duct papilloma excised from the breast

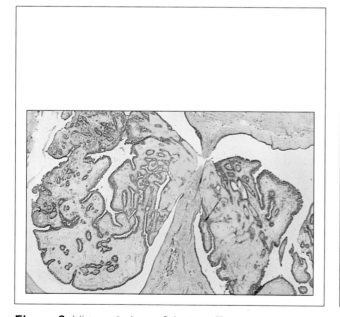

Figure 2 Histopathology of duct papilloma

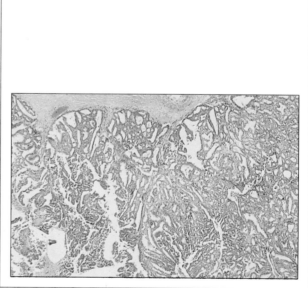

Figure 3 Histopathology of intracystic duct papilloma

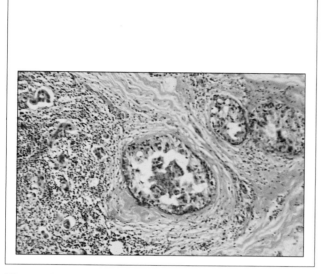

Figure 4 Histopathology of intraduct carcinoma with adjacent infiltrating polygonal carcinoma

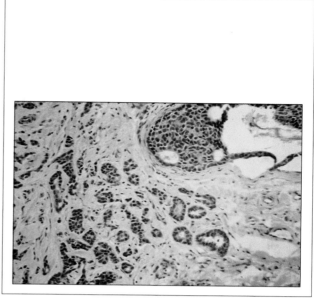

Figure 5 Histopathology of intraduct carcinoma infiltrating the breast tissue

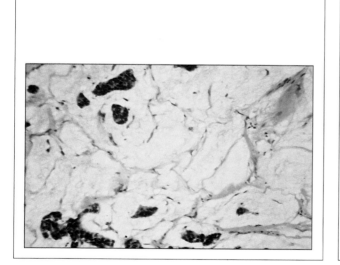

Figure 6 Histopathology showing the appearance of mucoid carcinoma of breast

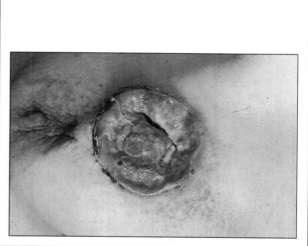

Figure 7 Carcinoma of the right breast, squamous cell variety. This is a rare malignant breast carcinoma

coalesce to form a localized tumour which continues to increase in size. Changes in the nipple occur, including elevation, deviation, retraction and ulceration. As the tumour enlarges, dimpling and redness are seen in the overlying skin. Oedema may be generalized causing the condition of 'peau d'orange'. In patients with advanced breast carcinoma, purple-red nodules develop in the skin of the breast, chest wall or the neck. These nodules in the breast skin may fuse into a large indurated area; in some patients the carcinoma has ulcerated through the skin when the patient is first seen.

By the lymphatics   The carcinoma invades the lymphatic vessels in the breast; the main periductal vessels run parallel with the larger and medium size ducts to the subareolar lymphatic plexus, which communicates with lymphatics in the surrounding skin. The perivascular lymphatic vessels accompany the branches of the axillary blood vessels and posteriorly anastomose with the lymph vessels in the deep fascia covering the pectoralis major muscle and then pass to the lymph nodes in the axilla. The lymph vessels in the central and inner parts of the breast accompany the branches of the internal mammary artery to the group of internal mammary lymph nodes.

The main lymph drainage from the breast is to the group of lymph nodes in the axilla which are usually the first to be affected by metastases. These are often present when the patient is first examined and in the more advanced tumours metastases are present in the axillary apical lymph nodes with a swelling in the subclavicular region. When the axillary lymph nodes are affected, further spread to the supraclavicular lymph nodes occurs and these become enlarged and hard.

Sometimes metastases develop in the lymph nodes in the opposite axilla. Metastases in the internal mammary lymph nodes may be present when the axillary lymph nodes are affected by usually they do not reach a large size. Occasionally they cause a swelling in the 2nd, 3rd or 4th intercostal space anteriorly at the lateral border of the sternum, the mass being fixed to the chest wall and the overlying skin being reddened.

In the late stages of breast carcinoma more distant lymph nodes in other parts of the body may contain metastases.

By the bloodstream   Carcinoma of the breast has a high malignant potential and distant metastases through the bloodstream are not infrequent in other viscera and tissues.

(1) *Lung metastases*   These may remain silent clinically although they are seen in chest radiograms and by CT scanning. Later they cause chronic cough and dyspnoea with chest pain and cyanosis. Blood-stained sputum may be present.

(2) *Pleural metastases*   These usually accompany pulmonary metastases. Pleuritic pain and a pleural effusion which varies in size may be the first evidence of pulmonary metastases.

(3) *Liver metastases*   The liver is frequently involved by metastases from breast carcinoma and becomes enlarged and nodular. Perihepatitis causes pain in the lower right chest and upper abdomen; jaundice may develop.

(4) *Bone metastases*   The skeleton is a very frequent site for breast carcinoma metastases. The spine, pelvic bones, femur, humerus, ribs and skull are often affected, but other bones may be involved and multiple metastases in several bones are frequently seen. These metastases cause pain which may be severe and referred, for example to the extremities; pain may be the first indication of osseous metastases and radiograms may be negative for several months. A bone scan is a valuable investigation for metastases. A pathological frac-

ture of the affected long bone may occur and vertebral body collapse is a serious complication.

Metabolic disturbances occur as a result of severe osteolysis causing hypercalcaemia, which threatens life unless treated and controlled.

(5) *Brain metastases*   These are not infrequent and the symptomatology simulates that of a primary brain tumour, causing headache, vomiting, disturbance of vision and convulsions.

Metastases are also found in other parts of the body, including the ovaries, adrenals and pituitary gland.

Histopathology
There are several varieties of breast carcinoma on histological examination.

Scirrhous carcinoma   This is a hard solid tumour which on transection has a whitish-grey colour with minute yellow flecks; the texture is hard and gritty. Microscopically there are both intraductal and infiltrative tumour of variable degrees. The malignant ducts are embedded in infiltrating carcinoma which shows various cell types and histological patterns. A scirrhous carcinoma frequently shows all stages of development and progresses from intraductal tumour to axillary lymph node metastases.

Mucoid carcinoma   This type of tumour is somewhat large and circumscribed and on transection there is a rounded or jelly-like tumour with few fibrous septa, and areas of haemorrhage are usually present; microscopically there are groups of carcinoma cells scattered about in a mucus matrix. The periphery is more cellular and may show the ingrowth of fibrovascular tissue. The infiltrating tumour in the breast tissue and the axillary lymph node metastases show a similar or more cellular mucoid appearance (Figure 6).

Squamous carcinoma   This is a rare malignant breast carcinoma. Microscopically all stages of metaplasia are present from columnar cell epithelium to marked keratinized carcinoma. The squamous stratified structure is present in the axillary lymph nodes and in recurrent tumours. These tumours are considered to be highly malignant (Figure 7).

Figures 8–10 illustrate other examples of carcinoma in the female breast.

Paget's disease of the nipple
In 1874 Sir James Paget, Sergeant Surgeon to Queen Victoria and Surgeon to the Royal Hospital of St. Bartholomew, London, gave the first description of this disease of the breast which bears his name! This disease is a chronic affection of the skin of the nipple and areola which is followed by the development of scirrhous carcinoma in the affected breast.

Paget studied 15 patients aged 40–60 or more years, in whom the disease commenced as an eruption of the nipple and areola. In the majority this had the appearance of a:

> florid, intensely red, raw surface, very finely granular, as if nearly the whole thickness of the epidermis were removed, like the surface of a very acute diffuse eczema, or like that of an acute balanitis. From such a surface, on the whole, or greater part, of the nipple and areola, there was always copious, clear, yellowish, viscid exudation. The sensations were commonly tingling, itching, and burning, but the malady was never attended by disturbance of the general health. I have never seen this form of eruption extend beyond the areola, and only once have seen it pass into a deeper ulceration of the skin after the manner of a rodent ulcer.

This is Paget's own clear description of this disease and he stated that in every patient he observed, breast cancer followed, usually after 1 year and at the most 2 years, in the affected breast. The malignant tumour always developed in the substance of the

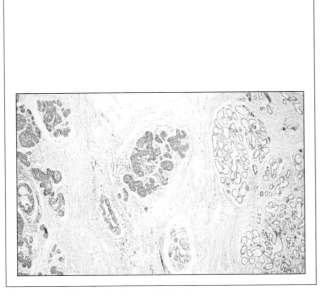

Figure 8 Histopathology of lobular carcinoma *in situ* and secretory change

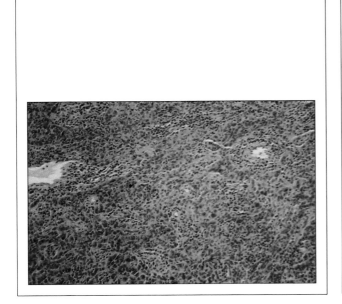

Figure 10 Histopathology showing appearance of medullary carcinoma of breast with lymphoid stroma

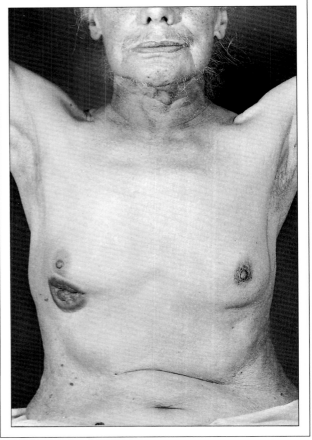

Figure 9 Carcinoma of the right breast – keloid variety

breast, beneath the diseased skin, or nearby, from which it was always separated by apparently healthy tissue. These tumours were no different from other forms of the disease.

Symptoms and signs
The first symptom noticed by the patient is usually itching or smarting of the nipple; the clothing near the breast becomes soiled and a crusted area or an erosion affects the nipple. A crack with a red granular base may be present in the nipple. Later the skin of the nipple and areola becomes red and moist with a serous discharge which may be blood-stained. The nipple finally becomes ulcerated and retracted (Figure 11). Palpation of the breast reveals a carcinoma present in any part of the organ. In another group of patients no tumour can be detected in the breast.

The regional lymph nodes are involved as in other varieties of breast carcinoma and there may be evidence of more extensive metastases. A mammogram may show the appearance of a carcinoma in the breast.

Paget's disease of the nipple also occurs, although rarely, in the male breast.

Diagnosis
It must be realized that these relatively small changes in the nipple and areola are the visible signs of breast carcinoma so that they are not mistaken and treated as eczema or dermatitis. The presence of a carcinoma in the breast should be assumed and confirmed by biopsy and histopathology (Figure 12).

Treatment
The stage of disease is assessed and the treatment is carried out as for other varieties of breast carcinoma.

Carcinoma of the breast and retinoblastoma of the eye
Retinoblastoma which arises in the pars optica retinae is a rare and highly malignant tumour in children of both sexes in very early life. There is an important hereditary influence and the offspring of patients who survive are at greater risk to develop this serious disease.

A female patient who had survived after excision of a retinoblastoma developed breast carcinoma 37 years later. This association is very rare and her family history is important.

Case record   A female aged 40 years was referred for assessment following treatment in another country. At the age of 3 months her right eye had been removed for a retinoblastoma. She discerned a lump in her left breast 37 years later, confirmed by biopsy as a carcinoma, and a left modified radical mastectomy was performed. Histopathology showed an infiltrating duct carcinoma with axillary lymph node metastases. Chemotherapy was given for 6 months followed by radiotherapy for 31 days. Tamoxifen was then given and continued. Clinical examination revealed no local or metastatic disease.

The patient's mother, who was aged 58 years, had undergone a radical mastectomy for breast carcinoma at the age of 44 years and was well 14 years later. Her father was alive aged 60 years following treatment for skin cancer of the face. She had one sister and two brothers alive and well. Her paternal grandmother had died with cancer of the stomach. Her maternal grandmother had died aged 90 years of old age but no cancer, and her maternal grandfather had died aged 69 years with multiple sclerosis. A maternal aunt had bilateral breast carcinoma and had metastases at the age of 52 years.

Bilateral carcinoma of the breast
A patient treated for carcinoma in one breast is at a high risk for the subsequent development of a new primary carcinoma in the remaining breast.

Case record   An unmarried female aged 46 years was referred with a carcinoma measuring 2 cm in diameter above the nipple in the left breast. A left radical mastectomy was performed followed by radiotherapy. Histopathology showed an intraduct carcinoma with early infiltration of the perivascular lymphatics. The remaining breast tissue showed adenosis with occasional cyst formation. Metastases were present in the anterior lymph node in the left axilla, but the apical lymph nodes were free of disease. The diagnosis was breast carcinoma, stage 2.

The patient developed a carcinoma 7 × 6 cm in the right breast 19 months later, confirmed by biopsy. A simple mastectomy with excision of the low right axillary lymph nodes was performed. Histopathology showed an intraduct breast carcinoma; there were no metastases in the axillary lymph nodes. A diagnosis of breast carcinoma, stage 1, was made.

This patient's family history is of interest. Her mother had a radical mastectomy for breast carcinoma aged 50 years and had died of cerebral thrombosis 18 years later, having had no recurrent or metastatic carcinoma. Two paternal aunts also had a radical mastectomy for breast carcinoma.

The patient was well 36 years after the first (left) radical mastectomy, with no recurrent or metastatic breast carcinoma.

Case record   A married female aged 39 years was referred with a carcinoma 4 cm in diameter in the upper, outer quadrant of the left breast and small lymph nodes in the left axilla. Carcinoma was confirmed by frozen section histopathology and a left radical mastectomy was performed. Histopathology showed a breast carcinoma with metastases in the left axillary lymph nodes; breast carcinoma, stage 2. A bilateral oophorectomy was performed, the patient being premenopausal.

The patient remained well until 20 years later when she developed a tumour in the upper, outer quadrant of the right breast, 5 cm in diameter. There were no palpable lymph nodes in the right axilla.

Excision biopsy showed the tumour to be a breast carcinoma 1.5 cm in diameter surrounded by fatty tissue. A modified right radical mastectomy was performed. Histopathology showed an invasive carcinoma and a microscopic focus of duct carcinoma. No metastases in the right axillary lymph nodes were found. Breast carcinoma, stage 1, was diagnosed.

The patient was well 23 years after the left radical mastectomy and bilateral oophorectomy and 3 years after the right modified radical mastectomy. It is of note that bilateral oophorectomy did not prevent the development of a carcinoma in the opposite breast 20 years later.

Case record   A female aged 64 years was referred from another country following local excision of a carcinoma 3 cm in diameter in the upper outer quadrant of the right breast. Histopathology showed a primary breast carcinoma composed of large polyhedral cells arranged as irregular groups in a fibroblastic stroma which displayed very heavy infiltration with lymphocytes and plasmacytes. Some of the lymphocytic aggregates had primitive reaction centres. This tumour was a medullary carcinoma with lymphoid stroma.

A right radical mastectomy was performed. Histopathology showed the changes of fat necrosis; metastatic polygonal carcinoma was present in two out of 18 right axillary lymph nodes. Postoperative radiotherapy was given to the scar and regional lymph node areas. The diagnosis was breast carcinoma, stage 2.

The patient remained well for 18 years, then discovered a lump in the upper, outer quadrant of her left breast and a left modified radical mastectomy was performed in another country. Histopathology showed a scirrhous carcinoma of the left breast infiltrating the breast tissue; six lymph nodes from the left axilla showed no metastases. Breast carcinoma, stage 1, was diagnosed.

The patient was well 19 years after the right radical mastectomy and postoperative radiotherapy for the stage 2 primary carcinoma and 1 year after the left modified radical mastectomy for the stage 1 primary carcinoma. There was no recurrent or metastatic breast carcinoma.

Advanced primary carcinoma of the breast

In past years, a number of patients with advanced primary carcinoma of the breast have been examined and treated. Spectacular results have been seen in patients treated by bilateral oophorectomy and bilateral adrenalectomy leading to complete regression of the disease, and the patients survived for many years. Our knowledge of hormonal control mechanisms and hormonal therapy is increasing but a full understanding of this important subject has not yet been reached. A significant development in the treatment of breast carcinoma has been the introduction of new synthetic hormones, especially Nolvadex (tamoxifen). Consequently, operations for endocrine ablation, including bilateral oophorectomy, bilateral adrenalectomy and hypophysectomy, are now performed less frequently.

The impressive results achieved by the manipulation of hormonal control mechanisms must never be forgotten, for they were historic milestones in the development of our knowledge about the causation and treatment of breast carcinoma. With continuing research, both clinical and laboratory, the hormonal control mechanisms will be clearly understood, so that they can be manipulated to prevent breast carcinoma or to reverse early carcinomatous changes in breast tissue and thus cure the disease. In the author's experience a reversal of advanced breast carcinoma has followed hormonal treatment; the reason why this occurs must be known.

It is fortunate that advanced primary carcinoma of the breast is seen infrequently today because of periodic medical examination, mammography and ultrasound investigation for the diagnosis of early breast disease. The following case histories are of individual interest and provide encouragement for the future.

Case record An unmarried female aged 44 years was referred with a carcinoma 3 cm in diameter in the upper, inner quadrant of the left breast and a hard mobile lymph node in the left axilla. Aspiration biopsy showed a carcinoma. A bilateral oophorectomy was performed and a course of radiotherapy was given to the left breast and regional lymph nodes.

The patient was well 14 years later, with no evidence of local or metastatic breast carcinoma.

Case record A female aged 59 years was referred with an advanced primary ulcerating carcinoma which involved the whole of the right breast (Figure 13). Histopathology showed a polygonal cell carcinoma, grade 3. The patient was treated initially by radiotherapy, with a tumour dose of 3100 R. A bilateral oophorectomy and a bilateral adrenalectomy were then performed. Postoperative radiotherapy was given with a tumour dose of 4500 R. In addition, fluoxymesterone and thyroxin were given.

A remarkable regression of the breast carcinoma occurred, with complete healing of the ulceration and disappearance of the massive breast carcinoma (Figure 14). The patient was well with no recurrent or metastatic breast carcinoma 11 years later. She died from a cerebral haemorrhage.

Case record A female aged 50 years was referred with disseminated carcinoma from a primary carcinoma in the left breast (Figure 15). Two years previously a swelling had developed in the right preauricular region; 9 months earlier a painless swelling had appeared above the inner end of the left clavicle and 4 months earlier she had noticed a large lump in her left breast and a small lump in the outer side of the left arm. Other similar lumps had appeared in the skin of the right shoulder, chest wall and right loin.

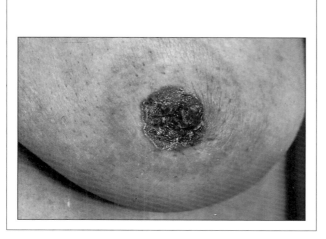

Figure 11 Female breast showing Paget's disease of the nipple

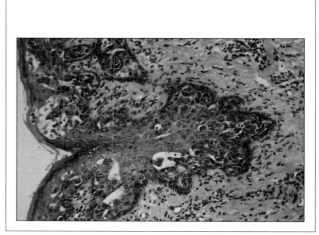

Figure 12 Female breast. Histopathology of Paget's disease of the nipple showing Paget's cells. There is hypertrophy of the prickle cell layers in and beyond the affected area; there is a broad zone of subepidermal chronic inflammatory cell infiltration

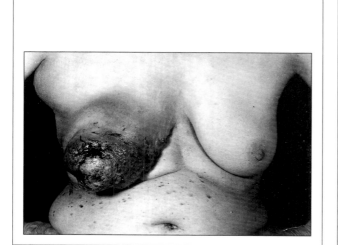

Figure 13 Female aged 59 years with an advanced ulcerating carcinoma of right breast treated with radiotherapy, bilateral oophorectomy and bilateral adrenalectomy

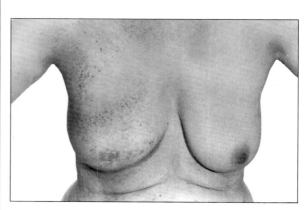

Figure 14 The same patient after treatment with radiotherapy, bilateral oophorectomy and bilateral adrenalectomy

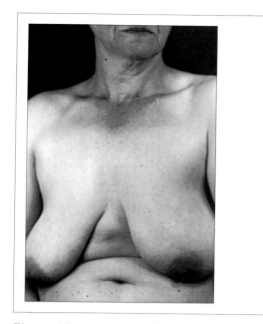

Figure 15 Female aged 50 years showing the enlarged left breast caused by a spheroidal cell carcinoma which had disseminated

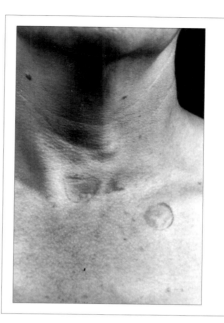

Figure 16 A skin metastasis below the left clavicle in the same patient

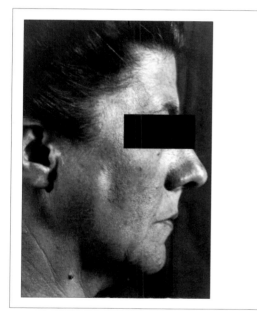

Figure 17 The right pre-auricular tumour in the same patient

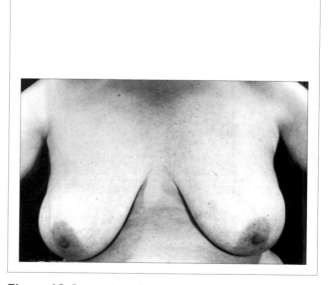

Figure 18 Regression of the primary breast carcinoma and of the skin metastasis below the left clavicle 1 year and 4 months after oophorectomy

Her menstrual periods had commenced at age 16 years; the cycle varied from 21 to 26 days with a duration of 7–8 days. During the last 2 years blood clots had been noticed in the menstrual discharge. This patient made the crucial statement that all the tumours increased in size prior to menstruation, and a decision was made to treat her by bilateral oophorectomy.

On clinical examination the following tumours were noted: right pre-auricular 3.4 × 2.2 cm; left supraclavicular 5 × 2.2 cm; and left breast, upper, inner quadrant, 3.5 cm in diameter attached to skin and fascia. Hard fixed lymph nodes in the left axilla and multiple metastatic tumours in the skin over the right shoulder, left arm, chest wall and right loin were present (Figures 16 and 17). The right breast and right axillar were normal and there was no abnormality in the abdomen. Radiograms of the chest, dorsal and lumbar spine and pelvis showed no metastases. A mild degree of anaemia was present.

A bilateral oophorectomy and excision biopsy of the skin tumour of the right shoulder were performed. Histopathology showed one ovary to be enlarged with a 2.5 × 2 cm cyst present containing watery fluid and it had a thin lining of luteal cells. The other ovary was of normal size, but there was a wide ill-defined zone of theca cell formation; otherwise it was normal. The skin nodule was a spheroidal cell carcinoma with cells arranged in compact groups and narrow cords, and there were isolated cells in the subcutis and deep layers of the dermis.

The postoperative results are of interest in that after 41 days the tumours were smaller and some skin tumours had disappeared (Figure 18). After 111 days the right pre-auricular tumour had disappeared, leaving a hollow area (Figure 19). The left breast carcinoma became very soft and smaller at 2.5 cm in diameter.

After 6 months there was a residual area of slight thickening in the left breast, a small lymph node in the left axilla and an area of thickening of skin in the left arm. A further 7 months later all the tumours had disappeared. The tissues of the left breast were soft, pliable, and normal; no lymph nodes were palpable in the left axilla, all the skin tumours had disappeared and the face was normal.

The patient remained well for 2 years and 6 months, when the right axillary lymph nodes enlarged and were excised. Histopathology showed anaplastic polyhedral carcinoma. The patient continued to be well until 3 years and 6 months after oophorectomy, then an enlarged right supraclavicular lymph node and small skin tumours appeared. These tumours regressed with methyltestosterone therapy and it was noted that the patient looked younger than formerly. There was no clinical evidence of primary or other disseminated breast carcinoma.

Five years and 6 months following oophorectomy a cyst 4 cm in diameter developed in the left breast. Later the patient's general condition began to deteriorate with osseous and soft tissue metastases present. Bilateral adrenalectomy was then performed. Histopathology of the adrenal glands showed no abnormality.

The disease continued to progress and because there had been such an impressive response to oophorectomy and androgen therapy it was agreed that a neurosurgeon should perform a hypophysectomy, but the patient died 2 days after the operation.

At autopsy, there was disseminated breast carcinoma in many organs, soft tissue and bones. Histopathology showed a highly cellular carcinoma in the left breast, invading the lymphatics and venules with local haemorrhages and areas of fibrosis.

The survival period of this patient with disseminated breast carcinoma from oophorectomy to death was 7 years and 6 months.

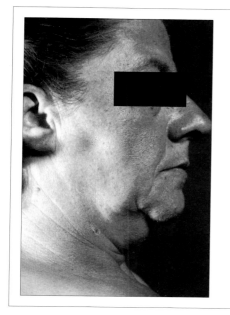

Figure 19 Complete regression of the right pre-auricular tumour after oophorectomy; this regression had occurred 1 year and 10 months following the operation

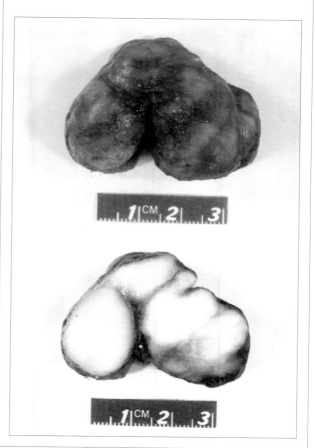

Figure 20 Female aged 23 years with a cystosarcoma phyllodes of the breast which is coarsely nodular, solid, lobulated, firm in consistency and whitish in colour

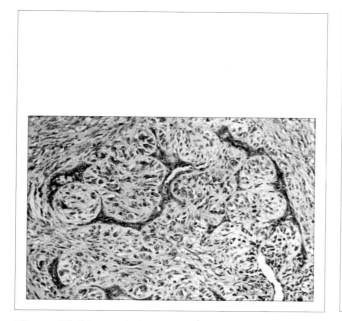

Figure 21 Histopathology of the cystosarcoma phyllodes shows the stromal and epithelial components of the tumour. Mitoses are frequent and there is a tendency to anaplasia. There are a few foci of lymphocytic infiltration

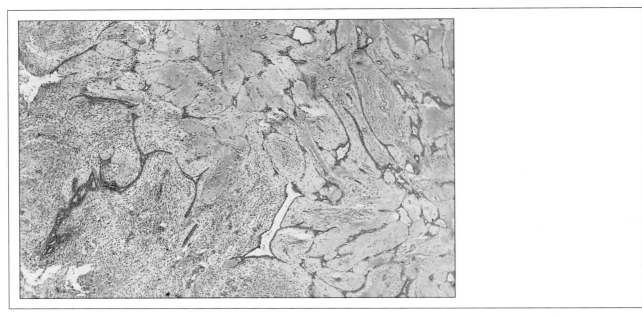

Figure 22 Fibrosarcoma arising in a giant fibroadenoma in the female breast showing the histopathology appearances, with fibroblast tissue

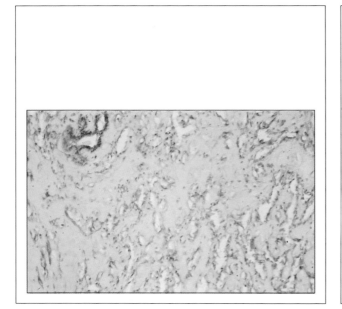

Figure 23 Haemangiosarcoma of the breast. The histopathology appearances

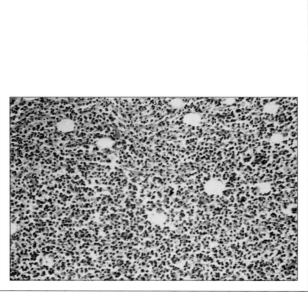

Figure 24 Lymphoma of the breast. Histopathology showing the typical appearance of this tumour

Cystosarcoma phyllodes of the breast

This breast tumour is rare and it represents less than 1% of all tumours of the female breast[2]. The tumour was described by Johannes Müller in 1838[3] so it is also known as Müller's tumour.

The association of cystosarcoma with carcinoma of the breast as illustrated by the following case history, is extremely rare.

Case record   A female aged 23 years was referred with a cystosarcoma phyllodes of the left breast which originally had been excised in another country and had recurred on two occasions. The recurrent tumour occupied the whole breast. The tumour was excised conserving the nipple and skin and a silicone breast prosthesis was inserted. The cosmetic result was excellent. Figures 20 and 21 show the macroscopic and histological appearances of the tumour.

One year later a recurrent tumour developed in the inner part of the left breast which was excised, conserving the prosthesis. A lump in the upper, inner quadrant of the right breast was also excised and on histopathology examination this showed the appearance of a highly malignant large cell carcinoma with areas of necrosis and very poor stromal reaction. Postoperative radiotherapy was given to both breasts, as well as a course of chemotherapy with melphalan for several months.

Eight months after radiotherapy a recurrent cystosarcoma phyllodes developed in the left breast; this was excised. Histopathology showed a higher degree of malignancy than previously. Further radiotherapy was given to the left breast.

Seven months later a small recurrent cystosarcoma phyllodes developed in the left breast immediately above the prosthesis, and a hard nodular tumour was present in the outer part of the right breast and a small nodule in the inner part near the nipple. A lymph node was palpable in the right axilla.

A right modified radical mastectomy was performed with removal of the silicone prosthesis in the left breast and excision of the recurrent tumour above it. Postoperative radiotherapy was given to the left upper anterior chest wall (the site of the small tumour) and to the lateral aspect of the scar in the right chest wall, the site of the large tumour. Histopathology of the right breast showed the tumour to be a cystosarcoma phyllodes; there were no metastases in the axillary lymph nodes and no recurrent carcinoma in the breast. The left chest wall tumour was a recurrent cystosarcoma phyllodes.

Eleven months later a recurrent tumour was excised from the inner end of the right mastectomy scar. Histopathology showed a recurrent cystosarcoma phyllodes.

The patient, who lived in another country, was alive 4 years and 9 months later, that is 11 years after the first cystosarcoma phyllodes was excised in the left breast.

Other sarcomas of the breast

All varieties of sarcoma of the breast are rare tumours in contradistinction to the frequency of carcinoma, and they usually affect the female, although a breast sarcoma can occur in the male. A sarcoma varies in its clinical appearance and the tumour may be quite large with haemorrhagic and necrotic areas. The consistency is solid or cystic. The tumour disseminates through the bloodstream and widespread metastases occur, chiefly in the lungs and bones. Lymph node metastases rarely occur except in lymphosarcoma. The following are examples of breast sarcoma.

Fibrosarcoma arising in a giant fibroadenoma

A breast sarcoma may develop from the stroma of a pre-existing fibroadenoma which is usually of the intracanalicular variety (Figure 22).

Haemangiosarcoma

This tumour is an even rarer variety of sarcoma of the breast. Clinically the haemangiosarcoma may reach a large size and a purplish discoloration of the overlying skin is present. The rate of increase in size varies from slow to rapid. Haematogenous metastases develop frequently. When skin involvement occurs there may be haemorrhage which can be severe and controlled with difficulty. Haemorrhage into the tumour causes a sudden increase in its size. The histopathology appearances are shown in Figure 23.

Lymphoma of breast

Lymphoma is rare in the breast and it may appear as a primary lesion or as part of generalized disease. In primary lymphoma there is a lump in the breast with evidence of infiltration into the breast tissue and the underlying muscle. The axillary lymph nodes may be involved, evidence then of more widespread disease. Figure 24 shows the histopathology appearance of breast lymphoma.

The breast is affected late in the progress of generalized lymphoma and becomes diffusely enlarged with infiltration and oedema of the overlying skin.

Sarcoma of breast followed by carcinoma

Case record   A female aged 33 years discovered a small swelling 1 cm in diameter in the upper, inner quadrant of her right breast. This tumour was excised in another country. Histopathology showed a poorly differentiated myxoid type of liposarcoma, with spindle cell differentiation and mitotic figures including abnormal forms which were numerous. Postoperative radiotherapy was administered to the scar area, with a total dose of 3500 R. There was no evidence of metastases. Her menstrual periods had commenced at age 12 years and the patient had taken the con-traceptive pill for the previous 2 years. She had 2 children aged 5 and 6 years who had been breast-fed for 6 weeks. The patient was examined 8 months following this treatment and no evidence of recurrent or metastatic disease was found. Fibroadenosis was noted in both breasts, especially in the upper half; there were no enlarged axillary lymph nodes.

Fourteen years and 4 months later the patient developed an infiltrating duct carcinoma in the right breast with metastases in the axillary lymph nodes. Right mastectomy with excision of the axillary lymph nodes was performed in another country.

THE MALE BREAST

The male breast is rarely affected by either benign or malignant tumours. When a malignant tumour does develop it is usually a carcinoma and its rarity in the male stands out in marked contrast to the frequency in females.

Gynaecomastia

This is not a tumour of the breast and is fairly uncommon. The condition usually develops about puberty and one or both breasts become enlarged to resemble the female breast. The breast is tender and in addition its size causes concern for the patient, to the extent that reduction mammoplasty may sometimes be requested (Figures 25 and 26).

An oestrogen-producing tumour of the adrenal cortex is extremely rare. In these patients gynaecomastia is a prominent symptom and is found in the majority.

Carcinoma

Carcinoma in the male breast when it does occur is usually unilateral (Figures 27 and 28) but very rarely both breasts are affected (Figures 29 and 30). Figure 31 shows the histopathology appearance of carcinoma of the male breast.

Symptoms and signs

The patient usually notices a lump in the breast which increases in size, sometimes at a rapid rate, to involve the overlying skin and ulceration occurs quickly. It

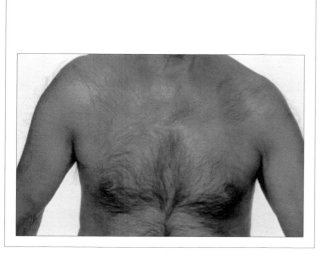

Figure 25 Male patient with bilateral gynaecomastia. There is uniform breast enlargement which resembles the female breast

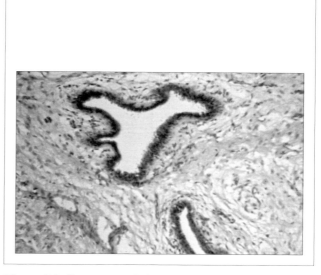

Figure 26 Gynaecomastia; histopathology appearance showing the marked stroma formation and resemblance to the virgin female breast

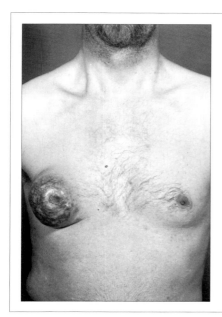

Figure 27 Male patient with a carcinoma of the right breast. A right mastectomy was performed with a wide skin excision and repair of the wound in the chest wall with an immediate skin graft

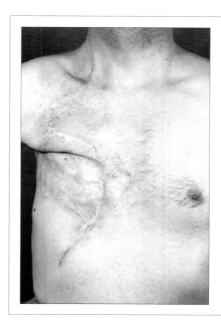

Figure 28 The healed wound following a right mastectomy for breast carcinoma

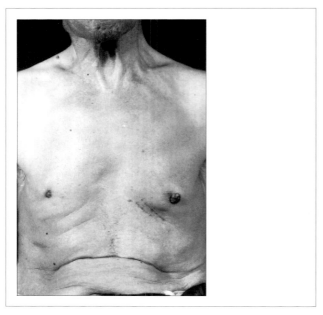

Figure 29 Male patient with bilateral carcinoma of the breasts before radiotherapy

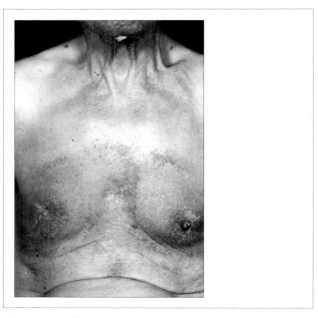

Figure 30 The same patient 5 months following radiotherapy showing the skin pigmentation over the treated area

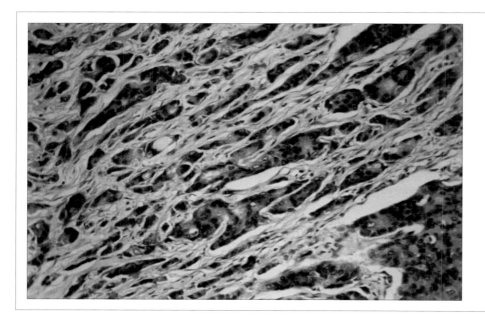

Figure 31 Carcinoma of male breast. Histopathology appearances

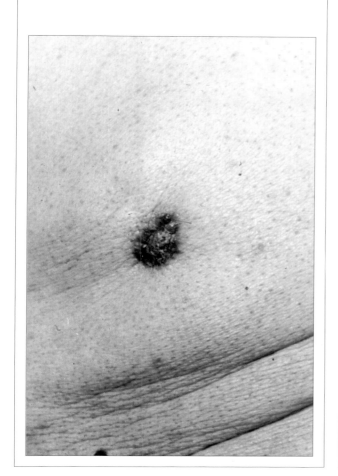

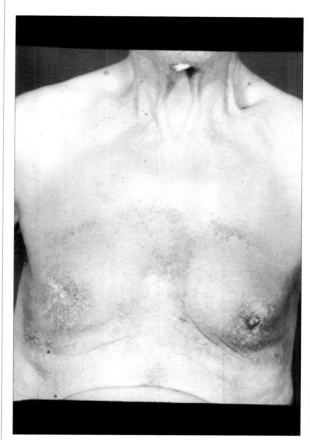

Figure 32 Male aged 78 years with bilateral Paget's disease of the nipple and bilateral breast carcinoma. The details of the nipple of one breast which resemble those of the disease in the female

Figure 33 The same patient following treatment with a full course of radiotherapy to both breasts; the appearances including the skin pigmentation following treatment. Note the enlargement of both breasts

seems that a discharge from the nipple is more frequent with breast carcinoma in men than in women. The length of history before advice is sought by men for treatment is longer than in women patients.

The carcinoma forms a hard lump in the centre of the breast which seen becomes fixed to the underlying pectoralis major fascia and muscle and to the overlying skin. The skin may be thin, reddened or ulcerated. The nipple is often retracted and may be ulcerated. The regional lymph nodes in the axilla on the side of the tumour are usually enlarged.

Spread of the disease

The spread of breast carcinoma in the male has the same pattern as in females. The tumour enlarges and invades contiguous tissues including the skin and pectoralis major fascia and muscle. Metastases occur in the regional lymph nodes and haematogenous metastases may also develop in the lungs and elsewhere.

Treatment

When the carcinoma is operable, that is it is not fixed to the chest wall, the axillary lymph nodes are mobile and there are no enlarged supraclavicular lymph nodes or other evidence of metastases, a modified radical mastectomy is performed. A much wider area of skin is excised than in the female patient and the resulting skin defect is repaired with a skin graft.

When the disease is inoperable a course of radiotherapy is given to the breast and regional lymph nodes. Local ulceration may heal with this treatment and there may be regression of the primary carcinoma.

Paget's disease of the nipple of the male breast

Paget's disease of the nipple is rare in the male.

Case record   A male aged 78 years was referred with soreness of both nipples and enlargement of the breasts. Examination showed the appearances of Paget's disease of the nipples and a tumour in each breast (Figure 32). There was no enlarged lymph nodes in the axillae or in the supraclavicular regions and chest radiograms showed no metastases. A biopsy was taken from each breast and histopathology showed the appearance of bilateral carcinoma arising in breast tissue.

A full course of radiotherapy was given to each breast (Figure 33). The carcinoma in each breast became flatter and softer in consistency.

REFERENCES

1. Paget, Sir J. (1874). On disease of the mammary areola preceding cancer of the mammary gland. *St. Barth. Hosp. Rep.*, **10**, 87–9
2. Dyer, N. H., Bridges, E. J. and Taylor, R. S. (1966). Cytosarcoma phyllodes. *Br. J. Surg.*, **53**, 450–5
3. Müller, J. (1838). *Uber den feieran Bau und die Forman der Frandhaften Geschwilste.* (Berlin: G. Reiner)

9

Tumours of the ovary

Tumours of the ovary are relatively frequent and are usually found in females between the ages of 40 and 60 years. Both benign and malignant tumours occur and amongst the former is the pseudomucinous cystadenoma, which may become malignant. There are several varieties of primary carcinoma and the prognosis is often serious because ovarian tumours situated deep in the pelvis do not cause characteristic symptoms, so patients in the early stages do not come for definitive treatment. Metastatic carcinoma occurs in the ovary, as described in Chapter 6.

BENIGN LEIOMYOMA

Case record   A female aged 26 consulted a gynaecologist on failing to become pregnant; it was found on pelvic examination that the uterus was much deflected to the left and there was some fixity around the left ovary. A salpingogram showed a unicornuate uterus with slight spill from the left Fallopian tube. As conception did not occur, a laparotomy was performed. The unicornuate uterus on the left side was confirmed; the left ovary was small and on section showed numerous retention cysts. The ovary was split and a wedge removed, and the ovary was repaired by sutures. There was no evidence of the uterus on the right side but a very long round ligament passed over to the right pelvic wall and the right ovary was suspended from this round ligament. A large smooth elongated tumour 20 × 7.5 cm was situated retroperitoneally on the side of the lumbar spine. A biopsy was attempted but bleeding occurred so this was impossible and nothing further was done.

The patient was then referred with this 'retroperitoneal haemorrhagic tumour'. She looked well. Abdominal examination showed tenderness in the right lower quadrant and a swelling 7.5 cm in diameter was felt. On radiological examination of the urinary tract by intravenous pyelogram, the left kidney appeared normal. The right kidney lay in the presacral region just to the right of the midline. The levicalyceal system opacified well; the uretic pelvis and calyces seemed a little distended and did not empty as well as on the left. There were 6 vertebrae of lumbar type, the last being partially sacralized.

The diagnosis was made of a right pelvic kidney which was functioning well and not hydronephrotic and the patient was kept under periodic observation. She continued well until 11 years later when she developed retention of urine; this was relieved by catheterization and normal micturition was restored. The retention recurred about a month later and was again relieved by catheterization. On both occasions the retention occurred on the 3rd day of menstruation (cycle length 31 days, duration 5 days).

On examination following these attacks of reten-

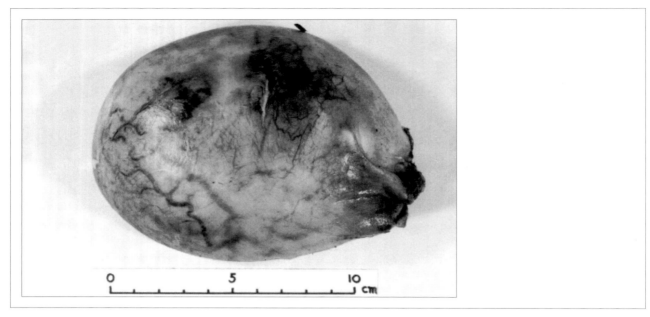

Figure 1 Female aged 37 years with a leiomyoma of the ovary which had caused complete retention of urine on two occasions on the 3rd day of menstruation; the specimen removed at laparotomy showing its thick capsule with a dense network of normal blood vessels

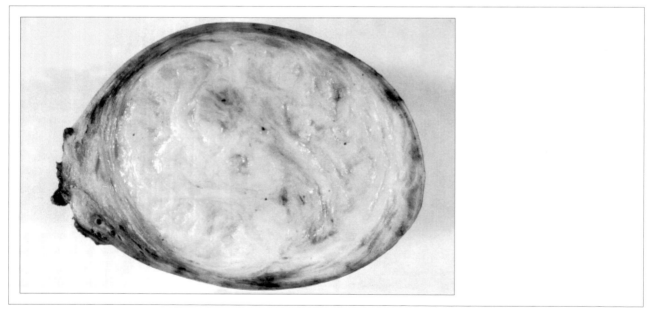

Figure 2 The leiomyoma of the ovary showing the appearance of the cut surface of greyish-pink with coarse trabeculation

tion a large swelling was found rising out of the pelvis to 8 cm above the symphysis pubis, more on the left side. A pyelogram showed that this swelling was not caused by a hydronephrosis of the right kidney.

A laparotomy was performed. A large round smooth tumour was firmly wedged in the pelvis; this was mobilized and removed. A rudimentary left ovary was conserved. The right kidney was situated in the right side of the upper pelvis and no gross abnormality was felt. The patient made a good recovery and was followed for a further 15 years with no more problems.

The left ovarian tumour weighed 680 g and measured 13 cm × 10 cm × 8.5 cm. The capsular blood vessels were prominent (Figure 1). The tumour was solid and rubbery in consistency; it was greyish-pink with coarse trabeculation on section. The lesion showed a thick fibrous capsule (Figure 2).

Histopathology showed the tumour to consist of fascicles of smooth muscle fibres with some interstitial connective tissue present. The thick capsule of the lesion contained a dense network of normal blood vessels. There was no evidence of cyst formation or malignancy. The appearances were those of an ovarian leiomyoma.

It is of note that the benign leiomyoma of the ovary had developed following a biopsy 11 years previously which had showed numerous retention cysts; at that operation the ovary had been split and sutured.

DYSGERMINOMA

Dysgerminoma is a special form of carcinoma of the ovary and is a similar tumour to seminoma of the testicle. The tumour is solid in consistency, firm and rubbery, and is well encapsulated during its early phase. On section is it greyish-pink or pink and homogeneous; areas of necrosis may be present.

Histopathology shows a matrix of connective tissue fibrils which contain clusters or columns of large uniform polyhedral cells or these cells may diffusely infiltrate the connective tissue. The cell nuclei are round, large and stain deeply. Frequent mitoses are seen and there are occasional giant cells in some areas. Collections of lymphocytes are present in the stroma.

Case record A female aged 14 years was referred with this history. She had had an abdominal tumour for 1 year. A laparotomy had been performed in another country; the left ovary had been removed with the primary tumour, and abnormal tissue in the region of the left kidney and a lymph node had been excised. Histopathology revealed the ovarian tumour to be composed of sheets, nests and cords of large round or polygonal pale-staining cells with large nuclei; some were hyperchromatic and others were vacuolated with prominent nucleoli and mitotic figures. They were separated by thick fibrous septa with lymphotic infiltration. The specimen from the region of the left kidney showed fibro-fatty tissue infiltrated by the same tumour tissue. No kidney tissue was seen. The lymph node showed chronic inflammation and no metastases. A diagnosis of dysgerminoma of the left ovary with spread to the region of the left kidney was made.

On examination the patient stated that she had had swelling of both lower limbs, worse on the left side, for 1 month, and her abdomen had become very distended; she had pain in both loins and had lost weight. The patient looked very ill and wasted and anaemic. The breasts were very underdeveloped. The abdomen was very distended with a large bulging tumour in the upper half, more marked on the left side. Large distended veins were present over a wide area of the abdomen and chest. Ascites peritonei was present, as was hepatomegaly. Rectal examination showed massive tumour involvement of the pelvis. There was marked oedema of the legs, worse on the left side.

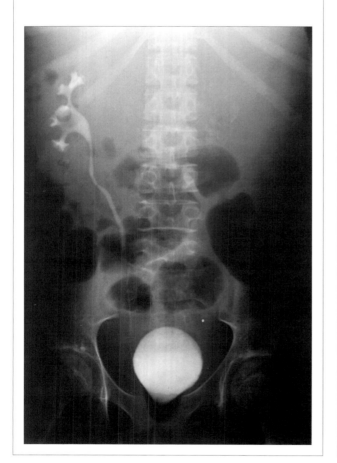

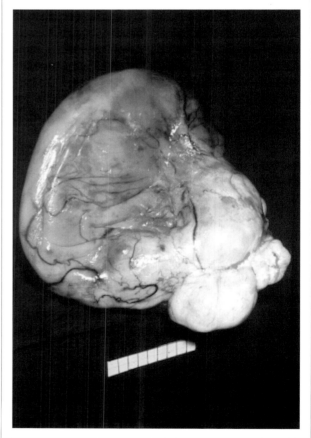

Figure 3 Female aged 14 years with a large abdominal and pelvic metastatic tumour from a primary dysgerminoma of the left ovary, which had caused a non-functioning left kidney. There was a remarkable regression of the tumour following radiotherapy and chemotherapy. Radiogram of an intravenous pyelography showing returning function in the left kidney

Figure 4 Serous cystadenocarcinoma of the ovary showing the unilocular cyst with numerous loculi studded with small sessile protuberances. A large part of the tumour is solid and greyish-white in appearance. The cystic area is vascular

The patient was fully investigated. Marrow cytology showed a hypoplastic appearance with macrophages relatively increased; malignant cells were not seen. There was severe anaemia and a raised erythrocyte sedimentation rate. Liver function tests and serum electrolytes were around normal levels. X-ray of the chest showed no metastases. Intravenous pyelography showed a normal right kidney and a non-functioning left kidney; the right kidney and proximal ureter were displaced laterally. Gonadotrophins were raised (501) equivalent to approximately 4–7 weeks gestation (this figure fell to 83 following tumour irradiation later); plasma oestradiol (58) was very low and consistent with ovarian failure.

The patient's general nutritional state was improved and 3 pints of packed red blood cells were given. A full course of radiotherapy to the whole abdomen and to the left upper para-aortic region was administered, with a total dose of 4950 R. There was a remarkable regression of the tumour and an intravenous pyelogram showed returning function in the left kidney (Figure 3). Her general condition markedly improved and a decision was made to give her a course of chemotherapy with chlorambucil.

The patient was examined 9 months later when she felt well and asymptomatic. No abdominal or pelvic tumour was found and there were no distended veins in the abdominal wall. She then returned to her own country and no further information was received.

This patient with massive metastatic abdominal and pelvic dysgerminoma of the ovary showed an impressive response to radiotherapy followed by chemotherapy. The regression of this tumour shows its radiosensitivity.

CYSTADENOCARCINOMA

This ovarian tumour is predominantly cystic and it may arise in the benign cystadenoma. There are two varieties, namely the *pseudomucinous* cystadenocarcinoma and the *serous* cystadenocarcinoma. The former is the least malignant of ovarian carcinomas. The serous variety is the most common of these tumours and may be unilocular or multilocular with numerous solid areas. The wall of the entire cyst or parts of the walls of loculi may be studded with sessile papillary protuberances. These may also appear on the external surface of the tumour (Figure 4).

Spread of disease

These ovarian carcinomas spread to the capsule of the ovary, which is invaded, and the tumour is disseminated to the peritoneum and omentum. The uterus and Fallopian tubes are involved by direct and lymphatic spread. The vagina is also implicated by direct tumour spread. Lymphatic spread occurs to the regional lymph nodes where metastases are formed. Ascites peritonei often develops and haematogenous metastases develop in the lungs, liver, bones and other sites.

Histopathology

The degree of cell differentiation varies in different tumours and in the same tumour and the cells usually conform to the serous or pseudomucinous type. The serous cystadenocarcinoma may present a predominantly anaplastic appearance.

Treatment

Treatment of carcinoma of the ovary when the disease is operable is by radical surgery and this includes removal of the affected and the opposite ovary with the uterus.

10

Sacrococcygeal tumours

A detailed and illustrated review of sacrococcygeal cysts and tumours was published in 1935 by the author[1]. It was stated there that the sacrococcygeal region is one of the commonest sites in the body for the occurrence of anomalies, cysts, sinuses and tumours of various kinds, but this is not surprising when we consider the complex nature of the development of this part of the body. There are changes which occur in the embryonic primitive streak: the formation and disappearance of the neurenteric canal and the postanal gut, and the formation of the terminal part of the intestinal tube by the development of the anal canal. Complicated changes also occur which are connected with the development of the genitourinary system. It seems possible, therefore, that any of these primitive structures may leave a relic of their existence and thereby make a significant contribution to that which has been designated as a histological potpourri.

SACROCOCCYGEAL TERATOMAS

The sacrococcygeal tumours described and illustrated in this chapter are very rare. These large tumours were studied in the museum of the Royal College of Surgeons of England and were drawn by a medical artist, the late S. M. Sewell, and published by kind permission of the College in the British Journal of Surgery.

A teratoma appears to be the commonest variety of tumour occurring in the sacrococcygeal region, but even so it is rare. The following illustrations are examples of sacrococcygeal teratomas.

Figure 1 shows a sacrococcygeal teratoma which was removed from the gluteal region. The greater part of the tumour consisted of a large multilocular smooth-walled cyst at its free end, and of other cysts at its superior extremity. The two larger cysts were filled with fatty material; amongst this were a few short dark hairs. Behind the largest of the upper cysts was a short blind coil of gut. On the posterior aspect of the tumour there were two areas of pigmented skin, and in the centre of the lower area was the orifice of a canal 2.5 cm in length.

The histopathology of the tumour is shown in Figures 2 and 3. The epithelium of the blind coil of gut was glandular and resembled gastric mucosa in parts; other portions showed intestinal type of epithelium. Beneath the epithelium there were small nodules of bone and cartilage and also a small lymph node.

Figure 4 shows a sacrococcygeal teratoma removed from a child born with a large tumour attached to the tip of the coccyx. The anus was rudimentary and faeces were passed through the vulva.

The specimen was half of a bi-lobed tumour

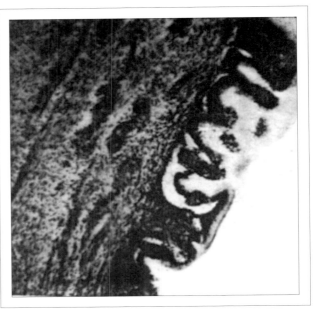

Figure 2 Histopathology of the sacrococcygeal teratoma showing epithelium composed of columnar cells resembling that of the large intestine. Numerous goblet cells are visible

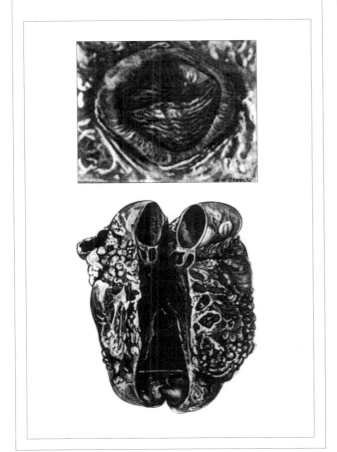

Figure 1 Sacrococcygeal teratoma (specimen in the museum of the Royal College of Surgeons of England); the upper illustration shows the cystic areas of the tumour, while the lower one shows the orifice of a canal

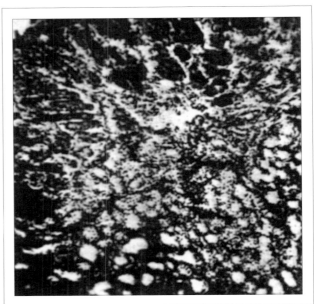

Figure 3 Histopathology of the sacrococcygeal teratoma showing glandular epithelium resembling gastric mucosa

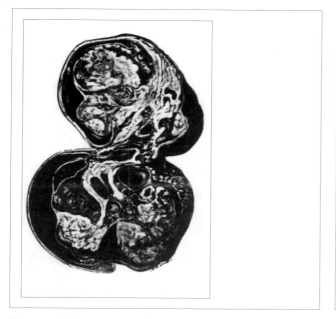

Figure 4 Sacrococcygeal teratoma (specimen in the museum of the Royal College of Surgeons of England)

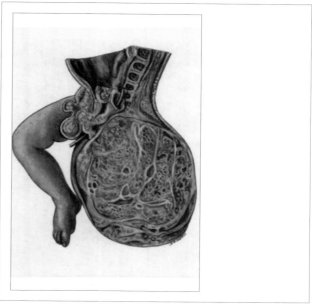

Figure 5 Sacrococcygeal teratoma (specimen in the museum of the Royal College of Surgeons of England)

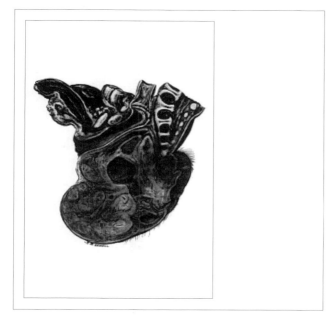

Figure 6 Sacrococcygeal teratoma from a premature child (specimen in the museum of the Royal College of Surgeons of England)

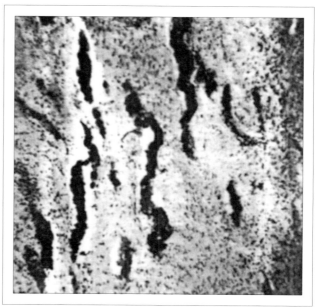

Figure 7 Histopathology of the sacrococcygeal teratoma showing well-defined processes of hyaline cartilage in the midst of supporting connective tissue

measuring 16 cm in its longest diameter. As displayed, it showed two cysts of about equal size consisting of skin with a thin proper wall adherent to it. A somewhat pedunculated solid growth projected into each cyst. The intracystic growth consisted of connective tissue in which lay an abundance of finely lobulated white fat. In the connective tissue there were embedded a few small islets of cartilage and bone (one of these is indicated in the lower segment by two black bristles). A certain number of well-defined, thin-walled cysts were distributed in the two tumours, especially about their bases of attachment. One of these cysts contained a few slender dark hairs.

Histopathologically, the main mass of the tumour consisted of simple adipose and connective tissue. The cysts were lined with columnar epithelium which was ciliated in parts. Some of these cysts were papilliferous, showing intestinal villi and crypts. In the fibrous tissue adjoining the crypts were sharply defined areas of neuroglia. Strands of instriped muscle ran in the course of some of the fibrous septa, but without any relation to the cystic spaces.

Figure 5 shows a tumour from an infant who was born with it and died at the age of 6 weeks. The specimen showed the right half of the lower part of the body of an infant. The rectum and lower part of the sacrum and coccyx were widely separated by a large oval tumour 14 cm in its chief vertical diameter. The tumour was everywhere sharply circumscribed and was minutely cystic throughout. It was imperfectly subdivided into lobes by strands of connective tissue.

Histopathology showed the tumour to be composed of spaces lined with cubical or columnar epithelium. In the intercystic partitions, branching plates of hyaline cartilage were present which had undergone ossification in places.

Figure 6 shows another sacrococcygeal teratoma, this one from a premature child born with this tumour. The specimen was a sagittal section of the lower part of the trunk of a premature child. Between the sacrum and coccyx and the rectum there was an ovoid tumour 7.5 cm in chief vertical diameter. The tumour was intimately connected with the skin and was of particularly soft consistency, though supported by somewhat coarse processes of connective tissue. It contained a few well-defined cysts, certain of which appeared to have ruptured on the posterior surface, and this had led to the production of external depressions. Immediately on the hinder wall of the rectum, below its middle, there was a small, minutely cystic area of glandular character; similar areas were to be found towards the posterior border of the tumour.

Histopathology (Figure 7) showed cystic areas lined with columnar epithelium. These cysts were dilated to form channels. The stroma contained nervous tissue in which large branching nerve cells were distributed. A few small well-defined processes of hyaline cartilage occurred in the midst of the supporting tissue (shown in the figure). Between the glandular elements were small groups and lines of fat cells.

It seems that these sacrococcygeal tumours are malformations. Further knowledge of their origin will be gained as experimental embryology continues to unravel the intricacies of the complex developmental processes and to throw new light on the growth centres of the body situated at the caudal extremity. It may be that these malformations will prove to be due to a faulty coherence of embryonal parts and a diminution of growth momentum[1].

REFERENCE

1. Raven, R. W. (1935). Sacrococcygeal cysts and tumours. *Br. J. Surg.*, **23**, 337–61

11

Tumours of the kidney and bladder

THE KIDNEY

The kidney is a relatively uncommon site for the occurrence of primary malignant tumours. On the other hand, metastases in the kidney from malignant tumours in other parts of the body are fairly frequent.

Hypernephroma

This tumour is the usual variety of malignant tumour of the kidney and it arises from the renal parenchyma. It varies considerably in size and may be quite enormous (Figure 1).

Appearance

The cut surface of the divided tumour has a characteristic variegated appearance with areas of different colours including white, red, brown and golden, caused by old or recent haemorrhage and lipoid infiltration in the tumour. The surface of the tumour is lobulated and largely defined, but with areas of infiltration into the substance of the kidney.

Histopathology

The microscopical appearances are variable in different tumours from well differentiated to non-differentiated cells. In the well differentiated tumours the cells are sharply defined with small dark nuclei and clear cytoplasm arranged as packed tubules or alveolar groups. In another group of tumours there are numbers of cysts where papillary proliferations of the lining project to almost fill the cavity. These papillary processes are covered with epithelium whose cells are finely granular. In some tumours there is a mixture of these types.

Methods of spread

The tumour spreads by direct extension into the surrounding kidney tissue. The renal capsule usually remains intact until the tumour reaches a large size, when invasion occurs into the perirenal fat. Direct extension occurs into the renal calyces and pelvis.

Spread also occurs in the lymphatics to form metastases in the para-aortic lymph nodes. Figure 2 shows metastases in supraclavicular lymph nodes. Important tumour dissemination takes place through the bloodstream when the renal vein or its main tributaries are filled with tumour. Haematogenous metastases occur in the lungs, liver, brain and elsewhere (Figure 3). A feature of this disease is the formation of a solitary metastasis. For example, a forequarter amputation for a solitary metastasis from a hypernephroma in the scapula has been performed by the author.

A patient was referred with a right hemiplegia which was caused by a hypernephroma metastasis in the left parietal lobe of his brain. The metastasis was accurately localized and treated with a course of radiotherapy. He was fully rehabilitated with the

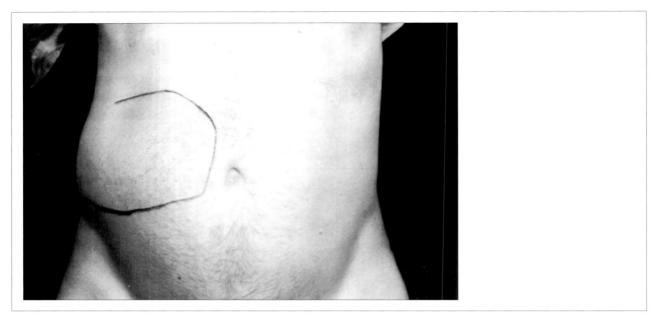

Figure 1 Male with an enormous hypernephroma of the right kidney

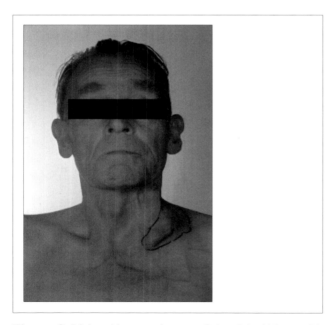

Figure 2 Male with a carcinoma of the right kidney with metastases in the left supraclavicular lymph nodes

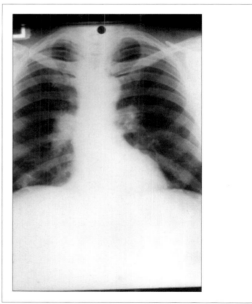

Figure 3 Male with a carcinoma of the right kidney with metastases in the chest shown in the radiogram

recovery of complete mobility of his right upper and lower extremities.

Local recurrence of a hypernephroma may occur in the scar following nephrectomy (Figures 4 and 5).

Leiomyosarcoma

A leiomyosarcoma of the kidney is a rare tumour with a very serious prognosis. The tumour spreads by direct extension into the adjacent kidney tissue and into the perirenal tissues. Spread also occurs by the lymphatics and metastases are formed in the renal and para-aortic lymph nodes. An important extension of the tumour occurs into the renal vein and haematogenous metastases develop in the lungs and liver.

Case record A male aged 48 years presented with a recurrent pain in his back, which occurred during the day or night, for 2 months. This pain became more pronounced in the left loin and radiated to the left testicle. Micturition was normal and there was no haematuria. He experienced no weight loss. The patient had had medical treatment for a duodenal ulcer for 15 years. On examination, tenderness was present in the left postrenal angle. An ill-defined swelling was palpated in the left upper abdomen, smooth and tender and not felt in the left loin. A chest X-ray showed no abnormality. A barium meal X-ray showed displacement of the stomach towards the midline by the tumour in the left upper abdominal quadrant. The pyelogram revealed a normal right kidney, ureter and bladder. The left kidney was enlarged with very little dye excretion. A left renal angiogram showed a mass in the hilum of the left kidney 10 cm in diameter with an extensive malignant circulation. The kidney was elevated by the tumour and showed no function; the tumour was circumscribed. Examination of the urine showed no abnormality.

Exploration revealed a large tumour of the left kidney with enlarged renal and para-aortic lymph nodes. The left renal vein was solid and very large; the left renal arteries were ligated and divided and the left ureter ligated and divided low in the pelvis. The left renal vein was then opened and it was found that the tumour extended throughout its full length; the tumour was extracted and the vein ligated and divided. The left kidney with the perirenal tissues was mobilized and removed. No metastases were found elsewhere in the peritoneal cavity.

Subsequently the patient developed a right empyema thoracis and a lung abscess which was drained 16 days later. He then made a good recovery. Postoperative radiotherapy was given to the left renal bed, left renal vein and para-aortic lymph node area with a tumour dose of 5000 R. Fourteen months later a CT scan showed multiple lung metastases and whole lung radiotherapy was given. Later metastases developed in the hilar region and both hepatic lobes; these were not controlled by chemotherapy. The patient died 2 years and 11 months after nephrectomy.

The appearance of the leiomyosarcoma of the kidney is shown in Figures 6–9. The left kidney measured 16 × 5.5 cm and weighed 1485 g with its fatty capsule and 850 g without it. The capsule was stripped off with some difficulty. There was a spherical tumour measuring 9 × 8 × 7.5 cm in the renal hilum which comprised the somewhat dilated renal pelvis. There were several seedlings of the tumour in the upper pole of the kidney. The renal vein was distended by a massive extension of the tumour. The tumour was soft to rubbery in consistency but solid, and on section was whitish with coarse trabeculation.

Sections of the tumour and its seedlings showed the features of a moderately differentiated leiomyosarcoma.

THE BLADDER

The majority of tumours in the bladder arise in the epithelium and range from the benign transitional cell

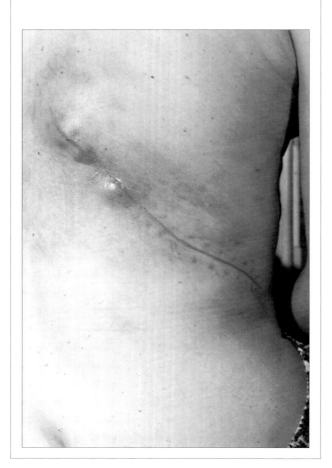

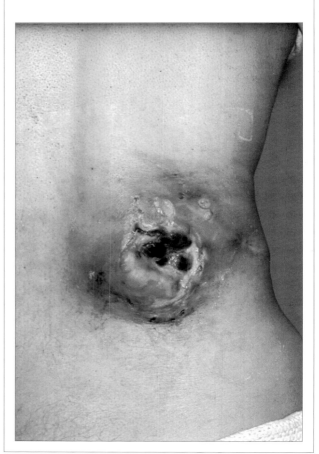

Figure 4 Male with a hypernephroma of the right kidney who developed recurrent hypernephroma in scar of nephrectomy and in the brain causing right hemiplegia

Figure 5 Carcinoma of kidney; recurrence in the right loin

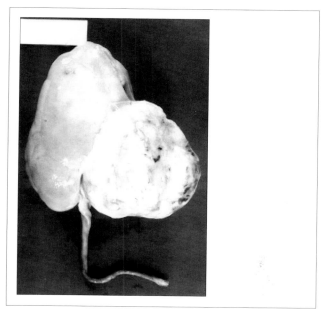

Figure 6 Leiomyosarcoma of the left kidney: external appearance

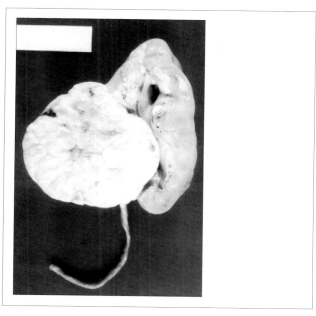

Figure 7 The cut surface appearance

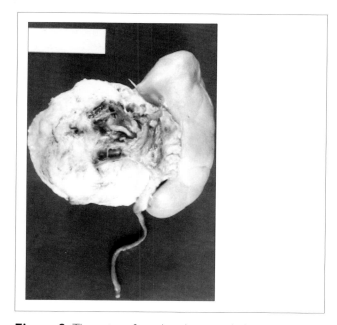

Figure 8 The cut surface showing vascularity

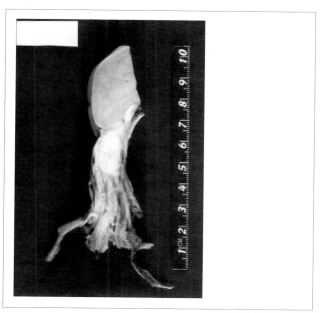

Figure 9 Invasion of renal vein and other blood vessels

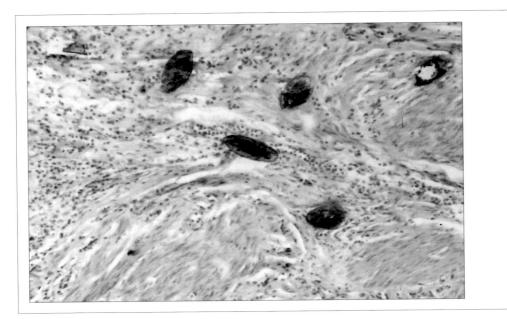

Figure 10 Histopathology of a carcinoma of the bladder associated with bilharziasis. The infection is seen clearly

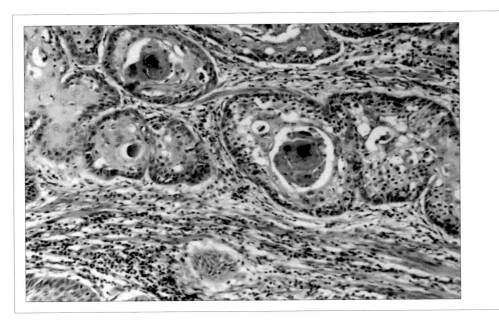

Figure 11 Another histopathology of a carcinoma of the bladder associated with bilharziasis. The infection is seen clearly

papilloma to the highly malignant invasive anaplastic carcinoma. Bladder tumours may be single or multiple. They occur at all ages and on the whole, males are affected more frequently than females. The carcinomas spread by direct extension in the bladder wall, which is later penetrated with involvement of the peritoneum. Direct extension occurs into the prostate, urethra and ureters. Spread takes place through the lymphatics causing metastases in the iliac and para-aortic lymph nodes either unilaterally or bilaterally. Metastases may also occur in the inguinal lymph nodes. Spread takes place in the bloodstream in the later stages of the disease when metastases develop in the liver, lungs and skeleton.

The bladder may be affected by direct spread of a malignant tumour in an adjacent organ such as the prostate, cervix uteri, urethra, rectum or colon.

Bilharziasis associated with bladder carcinoma

The frequency of malignant disease of the urinary bladder in Egypt is well known and has attracted considerable interest. This is attributed to the prevalence of bilharziasis in the urinary organs in Egyptians. The frequency of bladder cancer in Egypt when compared with African countries is related to the high endemicity and the frequency of bilharziasis in people who are obliged to be in contact repeatedly with infected water in the canals during their agricultural work. When patients are infected, cancer in the bladder occurs at an earlier average age than cancer in other organs in the same patients. Males are affected more frequently than females, possibly because females are less exposed to bilharziasis during their adolescence.

Monsa[1] stated that in the last 50 years, there has been a marked reduction in the morbidity and complications of bilharziasis including bladder cancer in areas where effective control of this infection has been established.

The histopathology of carcinoma of the bladder with bilharziasis is shown in Figures 10 and 11.

REFERENCE

1. Monsa, A. H. (1967). Bilharziasis and prevention of bladder cancer in Egypt. In Raven, R. W. and Roe, F. J. C. (eds.) *The Prevention of Cancer,* Ch. 38. (London: Butterworths)

12

Tumours of the male genital organs

TUMOURS OF THE TESTICLE

Primary malignant tumours of the testicle are relatively uncommon. There are two main tumours, namely *seminoma* and *teratoma*. These usually develop in patients who are young or in middle age although a teratoma occurs in patients a little younger than middle age. The tumour is usually unilateral; bilateral disease is extremely rare. In a few patients both seminomatous and teratomatous elements are present in the same testicle.

Familial incidence

It is doubtless a rather rare experience to encounter two members of the same family with a tumour of the testicle. The author has recorded this occurrence in two brothers[1].

Case record   A male aged 38 years complained of a painful swelling of the left testicle, which was increasing in size. Examination showed redness of the skin of the anterior aspect of the scrotum which was enlarged on the left side. The right testicle was normal. The left testicle was enlarged, hard and irregular. Testicular sensation was impaired but not absent, and a small hydrocele of the tunica vaginalis was present, which yielded blood on paracentesis. The spermatic cord was normal and the regional lymph nodes were not enlarged.

A left orchidectomy was performed with division of the spermatic cord at the internal abdominal ring. Postoperative radiotherapy was given to the para-aortic lymph nodes.

Histopathology showed the typical appearance of a seminoma of the testis; there were no teratomatous elements.

The patient made a good recovery and was well 5 months later.

This patient's brother was under the care of a surgeon at another hospital and his history follows.

Case record   A male aged 18 years underwent a right herniorrhaphy and 4 weeks later he noticed that his right testicle was enlarging. Six months later he was readmitted to hospital. On examination his right testicle was enlarged to the size of a cricket ball, hard and trilobed. A large hard lymph node was palpated immediately below the spine of the right pubic bone and there was a large mass in the right iliac fossa which was traced upwards along the midline to the liver.

This advanced disease of the testicle was inoperable and the patient died aged 19 years. No histopathology was available for this patient.

Malignant tumours in the undescended testicle

It is well recognized that there is a higher risk of a malignant tumour developing in an undescended testicle situated in the abdomen or in the inguinal region. This is considered to be due to the ectopic testicle being structurally and functionally abnormal, rather than to be caused by its actual position. Furthermore, a tumour may develop in the testicle many years following orchidopexy, probably due to the same factors.

Case record A male aged 48 years presented with this history. He had been born with an undescended left testicle and an orchidopexy had been performed at the age of 11 years. It had been noticed that his left testicle was atrophied when he was aged 17 years. Nine months prior to consultation his left testicle had begun to enlarge and had become hard in consistency, and 5 weeks earlier it was twice the size of his right testicle. Examination showed that the right testicle was high in the scrotum, smaller than normal, with normal sensation. The left testicle was much larger, 6.2 × 7.5 cm, solid and without sensation. No metastases were noted. Ultrasound examination showed a normal right testicle; in the upper half of the left testicle there was a heterogenous tumour 3.6 cm in diameter.

A left orchidectomy was performed. The histopathology specimen was described as that of a left orchidectomy with the spermatic cord measuring 7.0 cm in length and up to 2.5 cm across, with a cystic nodule at the site of the testicle measuring overall 4.0 × 3.0 × 3.5 cm. The cystic area with a diameter of 3.0 cm was partly filled by blood clot, while the wall was layered light brown, greyish-white and yellow tissue.

Sections showed a seminoma with occasional aggregates of lymphocytes and occasional multinucleate cells. The centre of the tumour was necrotic with cystic degeneration. No teratomatous tumour was identified. The adjacent testis was atrophic with prominent aggregates of Leydig cells. The tumour extended up to, but not through, the tunica albuginea, and the cut end of the spermatic cord was free from tumour.

Immunoperoxidase stain for HCG and a very occasional tumour cell was positive within the layer of necrotic seminoma lining the cystic space. (This is acceptable in seminomas and no teratomatous component was identified).

The patient was subsequently given a course of external beam irradiation to the iliac and para-aortic lymph node area and the retrocrural area on the affected side with a total dose of 3060 cGy.

The patient continued well 3 years after the operation and there was no recurrent or metastatic disease.

Seminoma

This tumour is a carcinoma which arises in the seminiferous tubules and is the commonest neoplasm of the testicle. There is some difficulty in distinguishing between the more anaplastic seminoma and the teratoma.

Appearance

The whole or part of the testicle is replaced by a homogenous tumour, firm and pinkish-grey, causing diffuse enlargement of the testicle, and it rarely penetrates the tunica albuginea. Sometimes small haemorrhagic areas are present and yellow necrotic areas are common.

Histopathology

The tumour is usually uniform in appearance with closely packed alveoli and trabeculae of large rounded or polygonal cells with clear cytoplasm and large central nuclei; mitoses are usually scanty. The tumour is divided into irregular lobules by connective tissue septa where there are lymphoid cells. Necrosis of tumour cells is common.

Methods of spread
Direct extension of the tumour may occur into the epididymis and spermatic cord. There is a high risk of metastases developing in the para-aortic lymph nodes. Late in the disease haematogenous metastases may occur in the lungs.

Mixed seminoma and teratoma
A small proportion of malignant tumours of the testicle show a mixture of seminoma and teratoma and there is no satisfactory reason for this particular combination.

Case record   A male aged 30 years had undergone a right orchidectomy for a tumour of his testis 19 months earlier and at the same time he had had a mass in the left hypochondrium, considered to be metastatic, and he had received a course of radiotherapy. The patient had subsequently been well and asymptomatic for 16 months, after which he had developed backache, and a radiogram had shown a lesion in the first lumbar vertebra. The abdominal mass had disappeared. The backache had persisted and 1 month earlier he had developed difficulty with micturition and a flaccid paraplegia due to a conus lesion at about the L1 spinal segment, some distance above the L1 vertebra. It was considered that there was intraspinal infiltration above the main bony level and the prominent spines of the D12 and L1 vertebrae were strongly suggestive of collapse of the vertebrae (see Figure 1). There were no metastases in the chest; the left lobe of the diaphragm was a little raised.

The patient came under the care of the author with paraplegia. Laminectomy was felt to be contraindicated. The patient received a course of high-voltage irradiation to the affected area of the spine with a tumour dose of 2050 R and a skin dose of 4000 R in 30 days. The paraplegia did not respond to this treatment and he died soon afterwards.

Histopathology of the tumour of the testicle showed the presence of a teratoma as well as a seminoma.

Teratoma
According to Willis, a teratoma of the testicle arises from dormant foci of pluripotential embryonic tissue, which have escaped the influence of primary organizers, so that tissues are produced that are foreign to the region in which they are growing. Growth with a rapid rate of tissue differentiation produces a benign cystic teratoma, but failure of differentiation with retention of the capacity for growth results in a malignant embryonic teratoma. Thus, teratomas of the testicle vary considerably in their malignant potential.

Appearance
The tumour usually is relatively small and since in most cases it occupies only part of the testicle, testicular size remains normal or is only slightly or moderately enlarged, unlike the case of a seminoma. The tunica albuginea is usually intact and on section it shows sheets of granular or smooth greyish-white tissue and not infrequently there are areas of haemorrhagic necrosis and large cysts. Occasionally fragments of cartilage or bone are present.

Histopathology
Teratomas show a marked variation of their component tissues, which are heterogenous and differ in the degree of differentiation. The more malignant tumours consist of poorly differentiated spheroidal and pleomorphic cells of variable size with marked mitosis which are arranged in irregular networks, diffuse sheets or in an imperfect glandular pattern. In parts of the tumour there is often a resemblance to a seminoma.

A variant is the choriocarcinoma, which is a very haemorrhagic and rapidly growing tumour composed of large undifferentiated cells. Some anaplastic seminomas which are very haemorrhagic and undifferentiated are also included in this particular group.

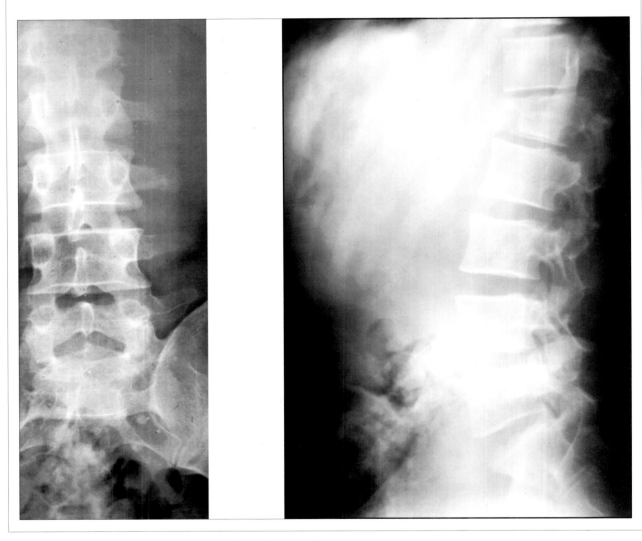

Figure 1 Male aged 30 years with a mixed seminoma and teratoma of the right testicle; radiogram of the spine showing collapse of the body of the first lumbar vertebra

Methods of spread

Teratomas of the testicle spread by the lymphatic system to form massive metastases in the iliac and para-aortic lymph nodes. In addition metastases occur in the mediastinal lymph nodes and even in the cervical lymph nodes. Spread by the bloodstream also occurs with the formation of metastases in the lungs and liver.

Symptomatology

In the main the symptoms and signs of a teratoma of the testicle are very similar to those caused by a seminoma. A teratoma is usually smaller in size, and usually it occupies only a part of the testicle.

Treatment

The treatment of a primary teratoma of the testicle is an orchidectomy with a postoperative course of radiotherapy to the iliac and para-aortic lymph nodes.

Case record A male aged 27 years presented with this history. One month previously a right orchidectomy had been performed in another country for a teratoma of the testicle. The patient had noticed the testicular swelling 5 months before the operation. Histopathology showed the appearance of a well differentiated teratoma of the testicle.

On examination, a hard fixed swelling in the lower half of the left side of the neck 6.5 × 5 cm in size was found. The left testicle was small and there were no other clinical signs. A chest radiogram showed a soft tissue mass in the left superior mediastinum above the aortic arch. A CT scan confirmed the large lymph node mass in the left superior mediastinum, and gross lymph node enlargement in the right para-aortic region. Multiple bilateral pulmonary metastases were present.

Combined radiotherapy and chemotherapy were instituted. Radiotherapy was given to the lymph nodes in the left cervical, para-aortic and pelvic regions. Chemotherapy included cis-platinum, vinblastine and bleomycin.

Biopsy of the left cervical lymph nodes was done and histopathology showed a relatively well differentiated teratoma of the testicle.

The patient continued under periodic review and assessment. Later a further course of radiotherapy was given to the neck, mediastinal and para-aortic areas. Chemotherapy continued in his own country and his condition was reviewed at regular intervals. Two years following radiotherapy and chemotherapy the patient felt very well and the disease was well stabilized. Chemotherapy continued with haematology monitoring. Four years and 5 months after his first treatments a hard swelling was felt in the left lower neck and was treated with radiotherapy, and chemotherapy continued.

The patient's general condition continued to be very satisfactory; he felt well and the disease appeared to be stabilized until 8 years and 6 months after his initial therapy, when the metastases in the left neck and para-aortic lymph nodes increased in size, with additional metastases in the lungs. Continuing chemotherapy was given. The patient developed impaired renal function so that chemotherapy was stopped 9 years after it was commenced. A chest surgeon and a urologist carried out a tumour 'debulking operation' through a right thoracolaparotomy.

At operation, a multicystic mass was found lying lateral to the paravertebral groove over the lower ribs; it was somewhat melanotic in colour due to a contained blood clot. Laterally the cyst extended through the intercostal space, bulging into the intervertebral foramen. There were many pulmonary metastases in all three lobes of the right lung, the largest being 2 cm in diameter lying on the posterior surface of the apical segment of the lower lobe. There was a large mass lying in the retroperitoneal position, obviously affecting the mesentery of the bowel. The paravertebral mass was excised. It ruptured on mobilization and old blood clot exuded. Excision was complete, sacrificing a single intercostal artery. Many of the pulmonary nodules were excised, but excision was deemed to be difficult and undesirable from this incision given the extent of the abdominal surgery. Nodules were therefore removed, one from the upper lobe, two from the middle lobe and ten from the lower lobe. Each of the lung defects was repaired with 3-0 Prolene.

In the abdomen the mass lay behind the inferior vena cava and in front of the aorta. It extended for the full length of the great vessels and out into the hilum of each kidney. Virtually all of this mass was removed in pieces. The only tumour not removed was the part wrapped around the left renal vein. Otherwise the abdomen was grossly clear at the end of the procedure.

Histopathology of the lung lesions was as follows: five had embryonal carcinoma; two had differentiated teratoma; two showed fibrous scarring and one was normal lung tissue. The abdominal mass was an extensively necrotic tumour, mostly of undifferentiated teratoma with some areas of intermediate malignant teratoma, with embryonal elements.

The patient made a satisfactory recovery from this major operation and returned to his own country under the care of his doctors there. He returned for review and received further chemotherapy 3 months after his operation. His general condition gradually deteriorated and he died 9 years after his first visit.

THE PENIS

The usual malignant tumour of the penis is a squamous cell carcinoma, but a small number of basal cell carcinomas have been described. These tumours resemble other carcinomas of the skin. The disease is relatively uncommon in the Western world. The most important single factor which influences its development is the practice of circumcision. Carcinoma of the penis is unknown in the Jewish race, where circumcision is performed on the 8th day after the child is born. It does occur, however, in others in whom this operation is performed later, chiefly between the ages of 3 and 15 years. In patients who develop penile carcinoma there is a high incidence of balanitis and phimosis.

Appearance
Carcinoma of the penis may be single or multiple and there are two main varieties. A *papillary* carcinoma involves the prepuce and the glans. Retraction of the prepuce becomes increasingly difficult. In other patients a *flat plaque* develops and infiltrates the outer aspect of the glans on the inner aspect of the prepuce or coronal sulcus and the region of the fraenum. Later ulceration occurs affecting the glans and the prepuce.

Histopathology
The majority of these tumours are well differentiated, keratinized squamous cell carcinomas. The widely infiltrating carcinomas are usually less well differentiated. Active mitosis is present in the tumour cells.

Methods of spread
Direct spread of the tumour occurs proximally in the subcutaneous tissues of the shaft of the penis. In the later stages of the disease the corpora cavernosa are invaded and there is marked distortion and destruction of the organ, and fistulae may be formed.

Spread by the lymphatics occurs early, especially in the infiltrating varieties and the poorly differentiated tumours. Metastases are formed in the inguinal and external iliac groups of lymph nodes.

Haematogenous metastases are uncommon, but in the late stages they may be present in the liver and lungs as well as in other sites.

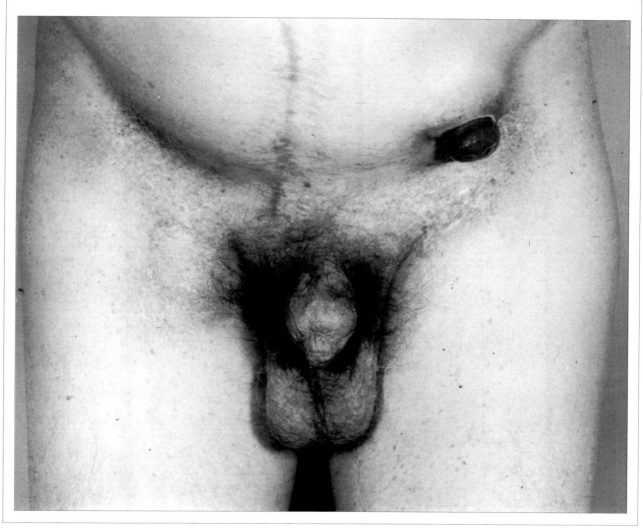

Figure 2 Male aged 57 years with a carcinoma of the distal end of the penis treated with radiotherapy and later by a partial amputation of the penis. Subsequently 7 years later he developed a carcinoma of the rectum treated by an abdominoperineal excision of the rectum. The figure shows penis and colostomy following these operations

Symptomatology

In the early stage of the disease when the prepuce can be retracted the patient complains of an ulcer or a wart on the glans penis and there may be a discharge. As the tumour increases in size the prepuce becomes more difficult to retract and a foul discharge occurs, as well as increasing difficulty of micturition. Gradually the malignant tumour ulcerates through the skin of the prepuce with increasing infiltration of the shaft of the penis. The inguinal lymph nodes may be enlarged due to infection or metastases.

Treatment

A carcinoma which is localized to the region of the prepuce and glans of the penis is usually treated first by a full course of radiotherapy. If regression and complete control do not result, a partial amputation of the penis is performed using a long dorsal skin flap, where the divided urethra is implanted to restore normal micturition.

When the carcinoma extends into the shaft of the penis to involve the urethra, corpora cavernosa and spongiosum, a total amputation of the penis is performed; the stump of the divided urethra is implanted in the skin of the perineum. For toilet reasons it is advisable to remove the scrotum and testicles because of the perineal urethra.

The treatment of the regional lymph nodes in the inguinal regions is carried out by the usual methods.

Case record   A male aged 57 years developed a carcinoma of the distal end of the penis. A full course of radiotherapy failed to control the carcinoma and a partial amputation of the penis was performed. He made a satisfactory recovery but 7 years later the patient developed a carcinoma of the rectum for which an abdominoperineal excision of the rectum was performed. He made a good recovery from this operation but 2 years and 3 months later he developed carcinoma metastases (Figure 2).

Case record   A middle-aged male presented with an advanced carcinoma of the penis with extensive infiltration of the corpora cavernosa and spongiosum. This caused increasing difficulty in micturition and finally complete retention of urine. On examination the patient's urinary bladder was distended up to the ensiform cartilage. There was an advanced carcinoma of the penis which extensively infiltrated the corpora cavernosa and spongiosum. There was no evidence of lymph node or other metastases.

This patient was admitted to hospital at once as an emergency and his urinary bladder was decompressed, thus relieving the complete retention of urine. Several days later a total amputation of the penis was performed and the urethral stump was implanted in the perineal skin. For toilet purposes the scrotum and testicles were removed, so that they did not hang over the urethra.

The patient made an excellent recovery from this operation. Normal micturition was re-established and the patient was alive and well 25 years after surgical treatment, and there was no recurrent or metastatic carcinoma.

REFERENCE

1. Raven, R. W. (1934). Tumours of the testis in two brothers. *Lancet*, **227**, 870–1

13

Tumours of the liver and spleen

BENIGN TUMOURS OF THE LIVER

Benign tumours of the liver are not uncommon and they may be mistaken for metastatic carcinoma.

Haemangioma

This tumour is found more frequently in the liver than in any other abdominal organ. It is usually small in size and occurs in the left lobe more often than the right lobe. When multiple tumours are present they cause nodularity of the liver. They are red-purple in colour, rarely protrude above the liver surface and are compressible unless calcification is present.

Adenoma

This tumour is not rare in the liver. It may be asymptomatic and discovered at laparotomy. The tumour may cause an upper abdominal swelling which compresses or displaces neighbouring structures and organs. The consistency varies from soft to hard, and the tumour may be single or multiple.

Connective tissue tumours

The tumours comprise fibroma, lipoma, leiomyoma and myxoma. They are usually small.

MALIGNANT TUMOURS OF THE LIVER

Primary carcinoma

There are two main varieties of primary carcinoma of the liver. *Hepatocellular carcinoma* arises in the liver cells; *cholangiocarcinoma* arises in the bile ducts. The disease is rare in the UK and in other countries of the Western world. It is more common in the Chinese and Javanese populations and in Africa, especially in the Bantu people. It is more common where liver cirrhosis and infestation with blenorchis sinensis are prevalent.

The disease can occur at any age, but mainly in adults, and it is more frequent in males than in females. The association of cirrhosis with primary carcinoma of the liver, especially of the hepatocellular variety, is well recognized (Figure 1).

Appearance

A primary carcinoma causes a bulky liver but its general shape is usually preserved. There may be multiple tumours present; most liver carcinomas are multifocal in origin. The right lobe is affected more often than the left lobe. In the hepatocellular variety, areas of necrosis and haemorrhage are frequent. A massive intraperitoneal haemorrhage may occur which can prove fatal. Early intrahepatic spread of the tumour is usual. The prognosis of primary liver carcinoma is very serious.

Metastatic liver tumours

In contrast with the rarity of primary carcinoma of the liver in the UK, the incidence of metastatic tumours is very high. Approximately one-half of the patients who

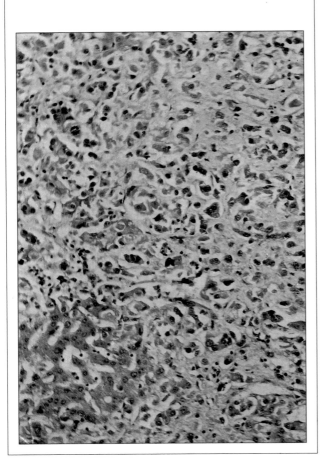

Figure 1 Histopathology showing the appearance of carcinoma in cirrhosis of the liver

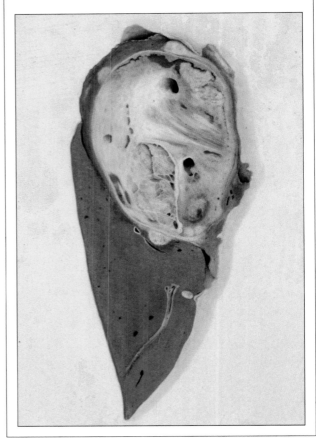

Figure 2 Metastasis in the liver from a primary kidney carcinoma

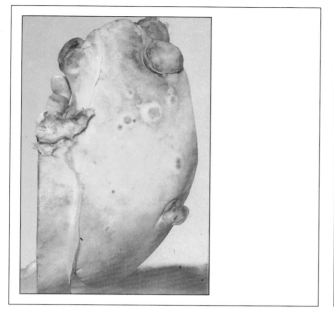

Figure 3 Metastases in the liver from a teratoma

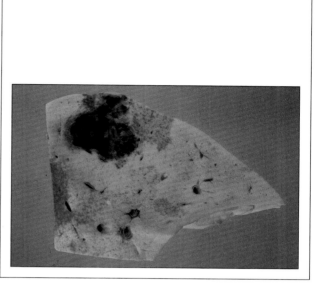

Figure 4 Metastases in the liver from a synovioma

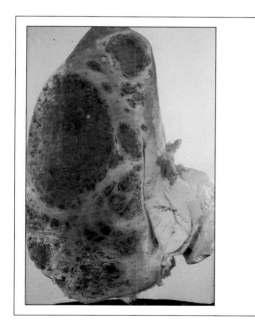

Figure 5 Metastases in the liver from a choriocarcinoma

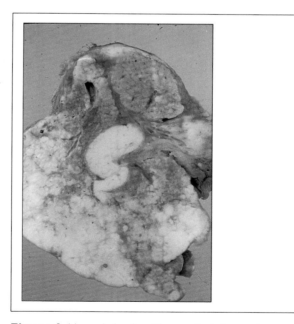

Figure 6 Liver cirrhosis with a metastatic carcinoma

die with malignant diseases have liver metastases. This vulnerability of the liver is caused by its position in relation to the portal and systemic circulations, its large size and the composition of its cellular components. Metastases develop from many varieties of malignant tumours, including carcinoma, especially of the alimentary tract and pancreas; of the uterus, breast, bronchus, kidney and adrenal glands; sarcoma of different varieties and sites; malignant melanoma; argentaffinoma; neuroblastoma; malignant lymphoma and teratoma.

Methods of spread

Portal vein dissemination   This is the main route for dissemination from the common sites of malignant tumours in the alimentary tract; tumours in other sites which are not connected with the portal system may spread to the liver by invading those viscera already connected, so that tumours in the ovary, prostate, bladder, kidneys and adrenals can metastasize to the liver.

It has been suggested that segregation of portal blood in the liver occurs; that is, that blood from different abdominal organs does not mix in the portal vein and has a lobar distribution, in that the left lobe of the liver receives a disproportionate amount from the superior mesenteric vein. Clinically one lobe of the liver is sometimes found to contain one or more metastases, while the other lobe appears free. This is an important observation in relation to partial hepatectomy. This problem was investigated by injecting 0.1 ml of ^{24}[Na] with an activity of 50 μC into a small tributary of the portal vein and the subsequent passage of radioactivity through the right lobe of the liver was recorded by a collimated scintillation counter placed directly over the centre of this lobe. The counter was then moved over the centre of the left lobe and the injection was repeated into a vein adjacent to the previous vein. These studies have not shown any marked asymmetry in the distribution of portal blood between the right and left lobes of the liver. It cannot be postulated, therefore, that a patient with a carcinoma in a certain part of the gastrointestinal tract is more likely to develop metastases in one lobe of the liver than the other[1].

Lymphatic dissemination   This is an uncommon route for liver metastases.

Direct extension   Spread by direct extension to the liver is common from a carcinoma of the hepatic and splenic flexures of the colon and the transverse colon, in addition to other neighbouring sites. The primary tumour becomes adherent to Glisson's capsule, an inflammatory reaction develops and malignant invasion occurs across this adherent area. Liver necrosis then follows with severe haemorrhage into the peritoneal cavity, lumen of the stomach or colon, and the patient presents for emergency treatment.

By the bloodstream   Metastases reach the liver via the hepatic artery from primary and secondary tumours in the lung. Spread of metastases within the liver is facilitated by its vascularity, and invasion occurs of the right or left main branches of the portal vein causing metastases in the corresponding lobe. When a large venous radical is invaded a wide liver segment is affected; invasion of a small venule causes metastases in a small area. One parent metastasis can thereby disseminate quickly throughout the liver.

Metastases in the liver invade the efferent hepatic veins, thereby entering the inferior vena cava, and are carried to the lungs. The liver acts as an intermediary for pulmonary metastases from primary tumours in the portal venous area.

Figures 2–6 are examples of metastatic tumours in the liver.

Liver lobectomy

The surgical excision of liver metastases has rightly attracted considerable attention for many decades with the objective of improving the prognosis of patients with these lethal diseases, which are so common. The development of hepatectomy operations during the 19th and 20th centuries is divided into two periods.

Segmental resections of the affected part of the liver were performed with intrahepatic ligation of the divided blood vessels, and considerable ingenuity can be discerned in the technique employed. The end-results of these operations in the 19th century were generally favourable for benign tumours, but much less satisfactory for malignant tumours. Local recurrence or generalized metastases frequently occurred several months after operation.

During the first 40 years of the 20th century, partial hepatectomy with intrahepatic ligation of the divided blood vessels was performed with great frequency.

The technique of left hepatic lobectomy with the extrahepatic ligation of the main blood vessels and bile duct of the lobe was described by the author[2]. Later this technique was applied to right hepatic lobectomy.

The following is the case record of the patient on whom the author performed his first left hepatic lobectomy for carcinoma metastasis.

Case record A female aged 52 years was referred with the following history. Six months previously she had had an attack of diarrhoea which had lasted about 2 weeks. This had recurred 2 weeks earlier and had been accompanied by a little bright red blood. She complained of flatulence but no abdominal pain; she had experienced some weight loss. Examination of the abdomen showed a swelling in the left of the epigastrium which was considered possibly to be a nodule in the left lobe of the liver. The descending colon was easily palpable. In the rectum, an ulcerating carcinoma surrounded the bowel lumen; the lower margin was 7.5 cm from the anal orifice and the tumour was somewhat fixed, especially anteriorly. Histopathology of the tumour biopsy showed a well differentiated adenocarcinoma of the rectum. The

biopsy had been taken from the edge of the tumour and the transition from normal mucosa to the neoplastic process was well shown.

An abdominoperineal excision of the rectum was performed. At laparotomy, the left lobe of the liver was found to be full of carcinoma metastases, with a tiny nodule abutting in the right lobe. The patient made an excellent recovery.

Four weeks later a left hepatic lobectomy was performed with extrahepatic ligation of the main blood vessels and bile duct of this lobe. The patient made an uninterrupted recovery from this operation (see Figure 7).

The pathological appearance of the left hepatic lobe was described as a portion of liver weighing 750 g. The hepatic tissue was largely replaced by massive greyish-white malignant deposits which imparted to the surface a typical umbilicated appearance. Histopathology sections showed a columnar cell adenocarcinoma, histologically of low malignancy.

The patient died 1 year and 7 months following hepatic lobectomy, presumably due to disseminated carcinoma.

Case record A female aged 47 had been treated surgically for a carcinoma of the rectum. She was referred with metastatic carcinoma in the right lobe of her liver. A right hepatic lobectomy was performed (see Figure 8).

The patient made an uninterrupted recovery from this operation. Two months later she was in good health, but further follow-up results are not known.

The pathology specimen consisted of the right lobe of the liver and the gall bladder. It weighed 880 g. The outer surface clearly showed a depressed nodule of tumour on the superior surface and other smaller nodules were also visible. On slicing there were two

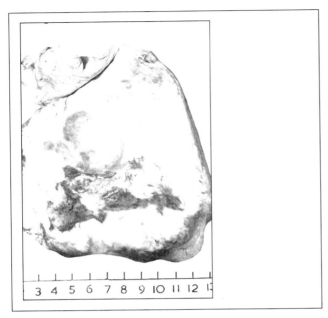

Figure 7 Female aged 52 with a carcinoma of the rectum treated by an abdominoperineal excision of the rectum. There were carcinoma metastases in the left lobe of the liver for which a left hepatic lobectomy was performed. Specimen of the left hepatic lobe showing metastatic carcinoma imparting a typical umbilicated appearance to the surface

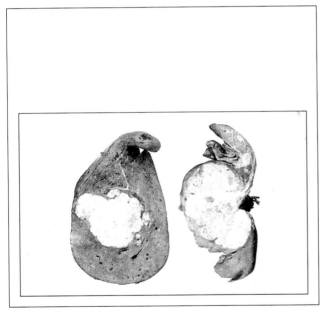

Figure 8 Female aged 47 years with a previous carcinoma of the rectum who was referred with metastatic carcinoma in the right lobe of the liver. A right hepatic lobectomy was performed. Specimen of the right hepatic lobe showing multiple carcinoma metastases

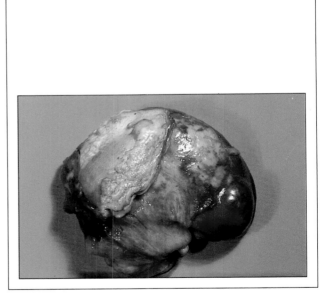

Figure 9 Female aged 48 years who had papillary adenocarcinoma of the Fallopian tubes and developed a large metastatic tumour involving the spleen, stomach fundus and left diaphragm. The appearances show part of the stomach wall attached to the splenic hilum; the spleen is enlarged and extensively infiltrated by tumour. A portion of the diaphragm is adherent to the upper pole of the spleen. Histopathology: papillary adenocarcinoma

large deposits of secondary tumour, each measuring approximately 7 cm in diameter, and one or two smaller similar deposits. Histopathology showed the liver to be widely infiltrated by a poorly differentiated adenocarcinoma consistent with a primary rectal origin. There was much necrosis and a good deal of surrounding fibrosis. Such liver as remained was congested and showed periportal inflammation with bile duct proliferation. The pathological diagnosis was liver: secondary carcinoma from the rectum.

The involvement of the liver by other tumours is described in chapters concerning these tumours.

THE SPLEEN

Primary malignant tumours in the spleen are very rare except for malignant lymphoma. On the other hand, metastases do occur in the spleen, especially carcinoma. Haematogenous metastases may develop from primary tumours in the bronchus, kidney, breast and ovary. The spleen may be affected by the direct extension of carcinoma in the stomach and the tail of the pancreas.

Case record   A female aged 48 years was referred from another country; she gave this history. Five years previously she had developed menorrhagia with uterine fibromyomas and pelvic pain. 4 years and 3 months earlier, a laparotomy had shown multiple uterine fibromyomas, bilateral tubo-ovarian masses and enlargement of both tubes, which were filled with fluid. Total hysterectomy with bilateral salpingo-oophorectomy had been performed. Histopathology had shown bilateral papillary carcinoma of the Fallopian tubes with one secondary deposit on the serosal surface of the uterus. There were multiple fibroids, and no metastases in lymph nodes.

When the patient was seen 4 years later, she had pain in the left loin which was present continuously and was sometimes sharp. She noticed flatulence and distension after food. On abdominal examination there was a little distension in the lower half of the abdomen; the spleen was palpable, three fingers' breadth below the left costal margin; the right kidney was palpable. An indefinite swelling was felt deep in the left lumbar region, possibly the left kidney or enlarged para-aortic lymph nodes. A swelling was felt in the epigastrium with its long axis horizontal and this seemed unconnected with the liver, which was not enlarged. No abnormality was felt in the pelvis. Investigations showed normal kidneys. X-ray with a barium meal showed a large mass completely obliterating the stomach fundus with the appearance of a neoplasm. Histopathology review showed papillary adenocarcinoma which appeared to arise from the epithelium of the Fallopian tube in one of the sections examined.

The abdomen and left chest were surgically explored by a left thoraco-abdominal incision, and a large malignant tumour in the upper left abdomen was found involving the stomach fundus and spleen and invading the diaphragm. The mediastinal, local mesenteric and coeliac lymph nodes were enlarged. No abnormality was found in the liver, pancreas, kidneys, intestines or pelvis. The tumour was removed *en bloc* including part of the left lobe of the diaphragm, the spleen, fundus of the stomach, part of the greater omentum and most of the lesser omentum. The stomach was reconstructed. There were outlying inoperable tumour deposits.

The patient made an uninterrupted recovery. A postoperative course of radiotherapy was given to the region of the left diaphragm and upper abdomen with a total dose of 4288 R.

The pathological specimen included the stomach fundus, spleen, omentum and part of the diaphragm (Figure 9), as well as part of the stomach wall 7 × 3.5 cm, to which was attached the hilum of the spleen. The spleen was enlarged and extensively infiltrated by tumour; it measured 14 × 7 × 5 cm.

Adherent to the upper pole of the spleen was a portion of diaphragm 8 × 7 cm whose pleural surface was studded with tumour nodules. Hemisection of the whole specimen showed a central area of necrosis surrounded by tumour. The spleen formed a narrow rim around the periphery.

Histopathology sections of the tumour showed a papillary adenocarcinoma whose appearance was consistent with origin in the ovary. Much of the central part of the tumour was necrotic; tumour infiltration of the spleen and diaphragm was extensive.

The patient returned to her own country for careful follow-up; an enlarged left supraclavicular lymph node was noted prior to her departure. Six months later the enlarged cervical nodes were treated with a course of radiotherapy with good regression. Her general condition remained satisfactory. Radiotherapy was also given to the left upper parasternal region, where a swelling had appeared, and this regressed satisfactorily.

The patient developed lung metastases 1 year and 5 months after the second operation and was treated with chemotherapy in her own country with improvement. No further follow-up reports were received.

REFERENCES

1. Raven, R. W. (1957). Liver surgery in relation to diseases of the colon and rectum. *Proc. R. Soc. Med.,* **50**, 775–86 (Section of Proctology 25–36)

2. Raven, R. W. (1949). *Partial hepatectomy.* Br. J. Surg., **36**, 397–401

14

Tumours of the thyroid and parathyroid glands

THE THYROID GLAND

Malignant tumours of the thyroid gland are not frequent and carcinoma is the common variety. As in other diseases of the thyroid gland, carcinoma is much commoner in women than in men and the reason for this sexual difference remains unknown. Unlike many other varieties of carcinoma which occur in patients in older age groups, thyroid carcinoma is found in children and young adults in addition to older patients.

Carcinoma of the thyroid gland

There are three main varieties of thyroid carcinoma which differ in their malignant potential. Macroscopically there are no distinguishing features, but their histopathology appearances are different.

Papillary carcinoma This tumour is usually quite small and the consistency varies from soft to hard. Histopathology shows functioning follicles and branching vascular papillary stalks which are covered by large cuboidal or columnar cells, and mitotic figures are uncommon. The malignant potential is less than in follicular carcinoma.

Follicular carcinoma This variety of tumour seldom becomes large in size but is usually larger than papillary carcinoma when the patient is first seen. It is firm in consistency and progresses faster than papillary carcinoma. Histopathology shows it to be com-posed mainly of medium sized follicles, often irregular in outline. Often the follicles are uniformly small, with or without a lumen. Some of the larger follicles are functional and contain colloid. The follicular cells are larger than normal and vary considerably in size and shape; their nuclei are often enlarged and hyperchromatic with occasional mitoses.

Undifferentiated carcinoma This variety of thyroid carcinoma contains neither follicles nor papillary components, and usually has a more uniform cell type than the other varieties. The tumour occurs in patients of all age groups but most frequently in the elderly. Local tumour invasion occurs, as do widespread metastases. Histopathology shows a solid small-cell structure with undifferentiated cells arranged in sheets. A giant-cell variety has been described which occurs most frequently in aged patients. Occasionally in this group there is a group of solid tumours composed of sheets of uniformly large cells with vesicular nuclei, and they occur at all ages.

Spread of disease

Local spread within the thyroid gland is very variable with different tumours. In a later stage the overlying skin becomes attached and the thyroid gland becomes fixed following extracapsular spread of the disease. The recurrent laryngeal nerve and the cervi-

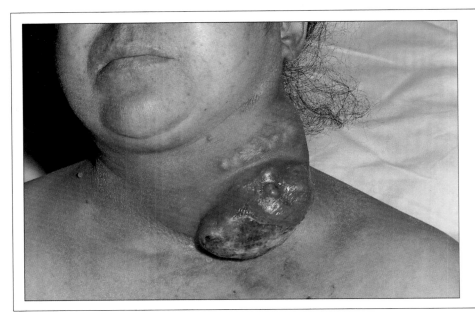

Figure 1 Female with a massive carcinoma of the thyroid gland which has fungated through the overlying skin of the neck with haemorrhagic areas; there are large metastases in the cervical lymph nodes

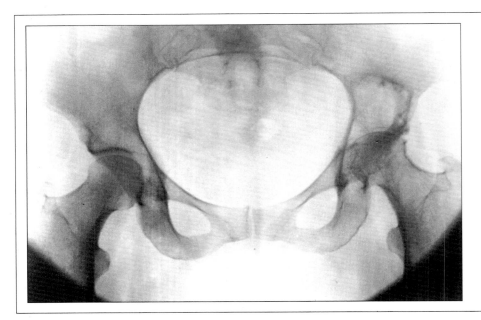

Figure 2 Female with a carcinoma of the thyroid gland showing a metastatic carcinoma in the left ilium involving the hip joint

cal sympathetic chain become involved in this local spread. In rare cases there is a massive carcinoma of the thyroid gland and fungation occurs through the skin of the neck; a patient with this advanced disease is illustrated in Figure 1.

Spread of the disease also occurs through the lymphatics to form metastases in the regional cervical lymph nodes in one or both sides of the neck. Haematogenous metastases develop in the lungs and bone and elsewhere. A metastasis involving a joint is somewhat rare and an illustration of a patient with a metastasis in the ilium affecting the hip joint is included (Figure 2).

Case record A female child aged 7 years was referred with an enlarged thyroid gland and enlarged bilateral cervical lymph nodes which had been present for 6 months. Another surgeon had examined the patient 4 months earlier and had found that she had enlarged tonsils; he had performed a tonsillectomy. The left cervical lymph nodes had remained enlarged 3 months and he had performed a biopsy of these nodes. Histopathology showed a metastatic papillary carcinoma of the thyroid gland.

On examination, a hard swelling of the left lobe and isthmus of the thyroid gland was found as well as palpable bilateral cervical lymph nodes (Figure 3). A total thyroidectomy was performed with a radical dissection of the left cervical lymph nodes; no abnormality was found in the right side of the neck. The left recurrent laryngeal nerve was separated from the carcinoma encircling it and marked with a metal clip for postoperative radiotherapy. A temporary tracheostomy healed spontaneously (Figure 4). A course of postoperative radiotherapy was given to the neck with a dosage of 500 R.

Histopathology showed the left lobe and isthmus of the thyroid gland to be replaced by a carcinoma; the bulk of the tumour consisted of a well differentiated adenocarcinoma. There was progressive loss of differentiation in some areas to sheets of simple polygonal cells with no acinar arrangement or colloid secretion. Metastases were present in the middle left deep cervical lymph nodes and in the prelaryngeal lymph nodes, but the highest and lowest cervical lymph nodes were tumour-free.

The patient developed normally and she was well with no recurrent or metastatic thyroid carcinoma 29 years after surgical treatment and radiotherapy. She was married and had two normal children.

Case record A female aged 15 years was referred from another country with an enlarged thyroid gland. The patient at age 5 years had developed a swelling in her neck which had caused dysphagia and dyspnoea; this had become worse 1 month previously. She had been seen by a physician in her country 6 months earlier and had been treated for hyperthyroidism.

On examination no exophthalmos or other evidence of thyrotoxicosis was found. The thyroid gland was enlarged, the right lobe larger than the left lobe, with marked enlargement of the isthmus; it was hard in consistency. The cervical lymph nodes were enlarged, especially on the right side where they extended higher in the neck; they were hard and mobile. A chest radiogram showed evidence of large numbers of very small metastases throughout both lungs.

A total thyroidectomy and a right radical cervical lymph node dissection as high as the mastoid process were performed. The primary thyroid tumour was adherent to the larynx and trachea and involved both recurrent laryngeal nerves, from which it was dissected leaving a small portion of tumour adherent to the right recurrent laryngeal nerve. A temporary tracheostomy was instituted because of the risk of laryngeal oedema. The patient made an excellent recovery and the tracheostomy healed spontaneously.

A course of postoperative radiotherapy was given

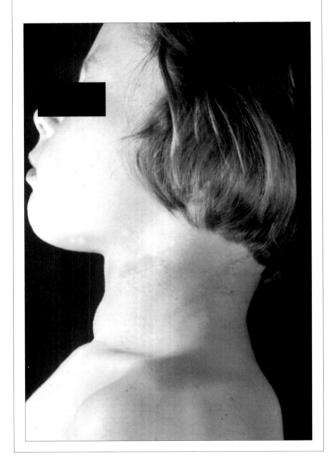

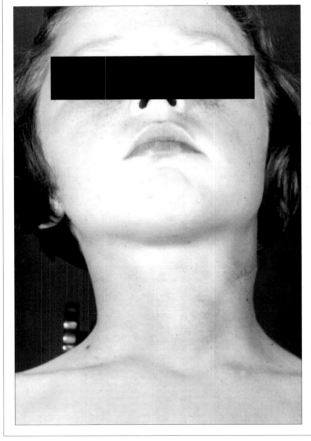

Figure 3 Female aged 7 years with an adenocarcinoma of the thyroid gland and metastases in the left cervical and the prelaryngeal lymph nodes

Figure 4 The healed neck after total thyroidectomy and left radical neck lymph node dissection. Patient alive with no recurrent or metastatic carcinoma 29 years later

to the neck. Radioactive iodine was administered for the lung metastases and thyroxine therapy was commenced. A left supraventricular lymph node was excised 4 months later.

Histopathology showed the appearance of a thyroid carcinoma of follicular type with colloid formation. The right cervical lymph nodes showed metastases of a similar nature and the left supraclavicular lymph node excised later showed similar metastases.

The patient was well and there was no evidence of recurrent or metastatic thyroid carcinoma 15 years following surgery, radiotherapy and radioactive iodine therapy. She was married and had given birth to three healthy children.

This case illustrates that, fortunately, a proportion of thyroid follicular carcinomas will take up therapeutic doses of radioactive iodine.

Lymphomas of the thyroid gland

Lymphomas may occur as primary disease in the thyroid gland. These include lymphosarcoma, reticulum cell sarcoma and Hodgkin's disease. Later in the disease lymphomas may affect the axillary, inguinal and para-aortic groups of lymph nodes. These tumours are relatively radiosensitive.

Lymphosarcoma

Lymphosarcoma of the thyroid gland usually has a poor prognosis.

Case record A female aged 50 years had developed thyrotoxicosis 12 years previously and she had been treated elsewhere with thiouracil and subsequently with iodine over a period of 10 years and she had developed severe hypothyroidism. On examination, enlargement of the thyroid gland, which was very hard in consistency throughout, was found. The cervical lymph nodes in the left posterior triangle were enlarged (Figure 5). Iodine uptake was normal. The diagnoses considered were thyroid carcinoma

and Hashimoto's disease. A total thyroidectomy was performed with removal of the enlarged cervical lymph nodes (Figure 6).

Histopathology showed the appearances of a lymphosarcoma which was poorly differentiated and diffusely infiltrating the thyroid gland. The cervical lymph nodes contained metastases.

Eight months following total thyroidectomy the patient developed a metastasis in the left inguinal lymph node which was excised. She was then treated with chlorambucil. The patient died with pulmonary metastases 21 months after thyroidectomy.

Lymphoma complicating pregnancy

It is rare to see a pregnant patient with a malignant lymphoma of the thyroid gland. A pregnant patient had developed an extensive tumour of the thyroid gland and she was referred for treatment. On examination an extensive tumour of the thyroid gland with a large retrosternal extension was found (Figure 7). A radical total thyroidectomy was performed, including the retrosternal extension; for this it was necessary to split the sternum to eradicate the whole tumour (Figure 8). Histopathological appearances were those of a malignant lymphoma.

TUMOURS OF THE PARATHYROID GLANDS

Tumours of the parathyroid glands, both benign and malignant, are very rare. Furthermore, it is considered that the majority of carcinomas of the parathyroid glands commence as adenomas.

Benign adenoma

Case record A male aged 20 years presented with this history. Three months previously he had experienced severe right abdominal pain, for which he had attended hospital, where appendicitis was suspected. His pain had ceased suddenly and 1 week later he had

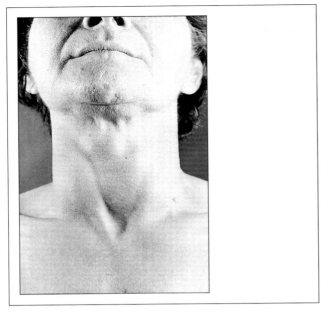

Figure 5 Female aged 50 years with a lymphosarcoma of the thyroid gland and metastases in the left cervical posterior lymph nodes, treated by total thyroidectomy with excision of the enlarged cervical lymph nodes

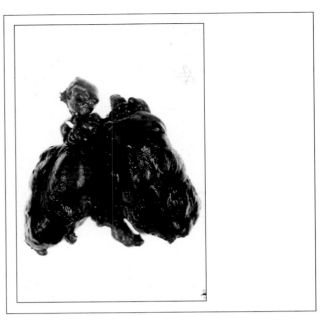

Figure 6 The specimen of lymphosarcoma removed. The thyroid gland is uniformly enlarged with the pyramidal lobe; white-yellow in colour

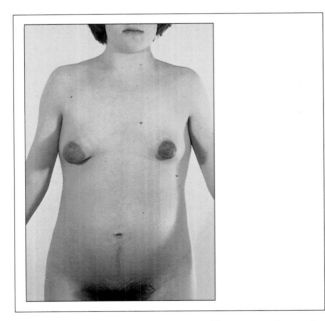

Figure 7 Female, who is pregnant, with an extensive malignant lymphoma of the thyroid gland including a large retrosternal extension

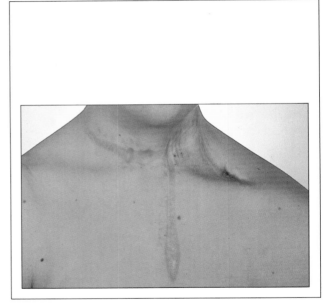

Figure 8 The same patient following radical total thyroidectomy and excision of a retrosternal extension for a malignant lymphoma of the thyroid gland showing the healed neck and sternal incisions

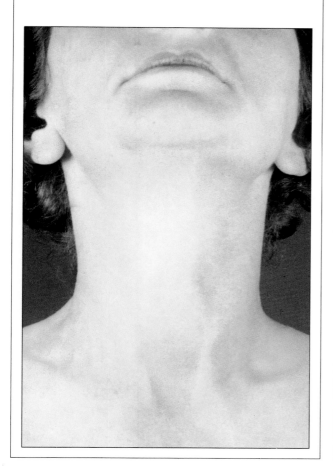

Figure 9 Female aged 47 years with an adenoma of the left parathyroid gland

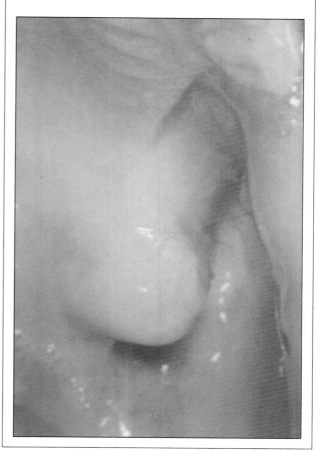

Figure 10 The tumour with a thin, transparent fibrous capsule, cream in colour and a slightly nodular surface

passed a calculus, which was half the size of a pea, in his urine. No haematuria was noted. The calculus was analysed and consisted of calcium. Blood chemistry showed the following results: calcium levels of 3.31, 3.23 and 3.20 nmol/l (normal range 2.25–2.62); phosphate levels of 0.72, 0.76 and 0.78 nmol/l (normal range 0.4–0.8). The 24-h excretion of urinary calcium was 14 nmol/l (normal < 7.5), with phosphates 41 nmol/l (normal 15–50). A recent IVP X-ray had been normal except for a small calculus present in the lower pole of the calyx of the left kidney. At the hospital the diagnosis was made of primary hyperparathyroidism, and exploration of the parathyroid glands was advised.

Clinical examination revealed no swelling of the thyroid or parathyroid glands in the neck and no other abnormality was felt. On the day of the operation the following were the results of serum analysis: alkaline phosphatase 17.1 units (normal 3.0–13.0); calcium 14.0 mg/100 ml (normal 9–11) equal to 350 mmol/l; inorganic phosphorus 3.4 mg/100 ml (normal 2.5–4.5) equal to 1.10 mmol/l.

Exploration of the neck showed a normal small thyroid gland. A parathyroid adenoma was identified attached to the posterior surface of the upper part of the right lobe of the thyroid gland, and it was excised. The patient made an excellent recovery.

Histopathology appearances were those of a parathyroid adenoma which was well encapsulated and composed of chief cells of the normal parathyroid gland, and oxyphil cells.

Postoperative blood chemistry a few days after the operation: calcium 10.2 mg/100 ml (normal 9.0–11.0), equal to 225 mmol/l; inorganic phosphorus 3.6 mg/100 ml (normal 2.5–4.5), equal to 1.16 mmol/l.

The patient was seen 8 months after the operation, when he was well. Blood chemistry showed: calcium 9.4 mg/100 ml (normal 9–11 mg); phosphorus 4.4 mg/100 ml (normal 2–5 mg).

The patient remained in good health and no abnormal clinical findings were present 13 years later. Blood chemistry showed: calcium 2.33 mmol/l (normal 2.05–2.60); inorganic phosphate 1.02 mmol/l (normal 0.64–1.60); alkaline phosphatase 55 IU (normal 39–117); urine analysis showed no crystals or other abnormality.

Case record A female aged 47 years gave this history. Two years earlier she had been admitted to another hospital with a tumour of the left upper jaw invading the antrum. This had been excised by a dental surgeon and the resultant oro-antral fistula had been closed by a mucosal flap with good healing. Histopathology showed the appearance of an 'osteoclastoma'. Nine months later the patient had been readmitted to the same hospital with a similar swelling involving the right antrum, orbital floor and the nasal wall. This had been removed and satisfactory healing had occurred. Histopathology showed the same appearance of an 'osteoclastoma'. Subsequently the serum calcium was 17%, which suggested that these giant cell tumours in this patient were due to hyperparathyroidism.

On examination, a globular swelling in the left side of the neck which was smooth and solid was found; the mass was 3 cm in diameter and moved with deglutition. The thyroid gland was not palpable and no enlarged lymph nodes were felt (Figure 9).

Investigations showed a serum calcium of 15.8 mg/100 ml; the repeat value was 16.4 mg/100 ml. On X-ray, there were signs of decalcification in the bones of the skull vault. A large cyst was present in the body of the right side of the mandible with marked thinning of the cortex, but without expansion. A similar, but smaller cyst was present in the posterior part of the left side of the mandible. A large cyst was present in the left maxilla passing across the teeth. Several smaller cysts were present in the region of the right maxillary antrum with probable involvement of the floor of the orbit. There was deviation of the trachea caused by a mass in the left side of the neck.

On surgical exploration of the neck, the thyroid gland was found to be normal in size and consistency. On the left side of the thyroid gland displacing it anteriorly there was a globular tumour, pale yellow and rubbery in consistency (Figure 10). This tumour had a capsule and was separate from the thyroid gland. The left inferior thyroid artery entered this capsule and then divided into branches. The left recurrent laryngeal nerve was stretched out over the inferomedial angle of the tumour. The lower left parathyroid gland was normal in size and consistency. The parathyroid adenoma was excised with the left lobe of the thyroid gland. The patient made an uneventful recovery.

The tumour weighed 27 g and comprised a tumour nodule $4 \times 3.5 \times 2.7$ cm, with a portion of thyroid tissue $3.8 \times 2.5 \times 1.5$ cm. The tumour was surrounded by a thin transparent fibrous capsule and its external surface was slightly nodular. The colour of the cut surface varied from cream to buff. The tumour was attached to the thyroid gland by delicate areolar connective tissue and a leash of thin-walled blood vessels.

Histopathology showed an adenoma composed of closely-packed, small polyhedral cells with spheroidal nuclei, scanty vacuolated pale-staining cytoplasm and ill-defined boundaries. The cells were arranged in large lobules, imperfectly separated by thin stromal septa. Numerous capillary blood vessels ramified through the lobules. In some fields the nuclei were rather irregular in size, shape and staining properties, but mitotic figures were not seen. The tumour cells resembled the 'chief' cells of the normal parathyroid gland. No eosinophilic or Wasserhelle cells could be found. The sections of the thyroid gland showed no abnormality. The diagnosis was that of a parathyroid gland adenoma.

Postoperative serum calcium values (preoperatively these had been 15.8 mg/100 ml and 16.4 mg/100 ml) were: immediate 10.5 mg/100 ml; 6 hours later, 9.6 mg 100 ml; and 24 hours later, 8.6 mg/100 ml.

Subsequently the serum calcium remained within normal limits. Alkaline phosphatase was 46 units/100 ml, electrolytes were normal and inorganic phosphorus was 2.6 mg/100 ml.

Carcinoma of the parathyroid glands

Carcinoma is a very rare tumour of the parathyroid glands and the majority are secretory, manifesting the general effects of the parathormone hormone. Parathyroid hyperfunction causes elevation of the patient's serum calcium with an increase in the excretion of urinary calcium, increased serum alkaline phosphatase, increased urinary phosphate excretion, decreased serum inorganic phosphorus and mobilization of the calcium in bone. These important biochemical changes cause severe symptoms and signs.

Symptomatology

Early symptoms are vague pains in various bones and joints. With the increased serum calcium, abdominal cramps and vomiting occur with lassitude, muscle weakness and weight loss. The osteoporosis leads to the formation of bone cysts including such locations as the jaws. Bone deformities and fractures may occur. Calcium is deposited in the cardiovascular and urinary systems so that polyuria, haematuria and renal failure occur. Calculi form in the kidneys and may be excreted if small, causing severe renal colic. Radiology may show calcification in the tumour in the neck or tracheal displacement, and renal calculi may be seen.

The non-secreting carcinoma causes few symptoms and signs until it has reached a large size, when a hard tumour is palpable in the neck. Local spread in the infrahyoid muscles and trachea causes dyspnoea and dysphagia from oesophageal pressure. The regional cervical lymph nodes may be enlarged, and late in the disease there may be metastases in the liver and lungs.

It is of note that the symptoms and signs of hyperparathyroidism described here are also caused by an adenoma of the parathyroid glands.

Spread of carcinoma of the parathyroid glands

Direct spread   Direct extension into the neck structures including the infrahyoid muscles, thyroid gland and the recurrent laryngeal nerve occurs. Large tumours may compress the carotid sheath and internal jugular vein.

Spread by lymphatics   This is an uncommon method but sometimes metastases occur in the cervical lymph nodes.

Spread by blood vessels   Metastases in distant organs are very rare but may occur in the lungs and liver.

Appearance of the carcinoma

The carcinoma is usually found to be attached to the posterior surface of a lobe of the thyroid gland outside the true capsule and in either side of the neck. The tumour is hard and nodular, reddish or greyish-brown and initially there is a well-defined capsule. Some tumours are cystic and others are haemorrhagic, and they vary in size.

Histopathology

Both secretory and non-secretory carcinomas resemble the structure of the normal parathyroid gland and its three types of cells are seen, the most frequent being the Wasserhelle water-clear cells, and sometimes there are scattered clumps of oxyphil cells. The cells may be arranged in solid masses, acini or trabeculae with a fibrous stroma. Mitotic figures are often absent except in the rapidly growing tumours, when there are giant cells, large nuclei and hyperchromatism, and marked vascularity may also be present.

Treatment

An adenoma of the parathyroid gland is excised with complete relief of the hypercalcaemia. Radical surgical excision is performed for the operable carcinoma; if the carcinoma is secretory, removal gives relief of the hypercalcaemia.

15

Tumours of the nervous system

Tumours develop in the nervous system as their primary site or occur as metastases from malignant tumours in other tissues and sites of the body. Metastatic tumours are quite common in the brain, where they cause serious complications. In the nervous system there are various tumours which are classified as benign on histopathological appearances but which cannot be removed completely and eventually cause complications and the death of the patient. These tumours include certain meningiomas, acoustic tumours and tumours of the pituitary gland.

TUMOURS OF THE BRAIN

Brain tumours occur at all ages but their type and characteristics differ in different age groups. Thus, in children tumours of the cerebellum are more common than tumours of the cerebral cortex; the reverse is true where adults are concerned. In children the commonest malignant tumour is the astrocytoma, which is often cystic. In adults various malignant tumours occur and have a predilection for different sites. Thus, various astrocytomas in adults occur in the cerebrum and usually are non-cystic. Meningiomas are commoner in later middle life and occur in other sites including the sella turcica and parasellar regions. Malignant brain tumours seldom cause a metastasis but they extend in the brain and affect neighbouring structures by direct infiltration or pressure effects. With a tumour in a cerebral hemisphere an initial adjustment is possible because of fluid in the ventricles and subarachnoid space, and the affected hemisphere is displaced toward the opposite side and downward. Later further adjustments become impossible and serious effects occur, including oedema of the brain.

No attempt in this chapter is made to describe the classification and different varieties of brain tumour nor their clinical manifestations and treatment. This is a large and intricate subject for the specialists in Neurology.

Metastatic brain tumours

Metastatic brain tumours may be single or multiple and may occur in any part of the brain. They are usually well defined and of homogeneous consistency, but necrosis and cyst formation are common. Occasionally haemorrhage into the tumour occurs and causes more severe symptoms.

The majority of brain metastases are carcinomas. Common primary sites are the lung in males and the breast in females. In patients with a lung carcinoma the intracranial metastases may cause the first symptoms of this disease. Hypernephromas of the kidney may metastasize to the brain (see also Chapter 11). Metastatic malignant melanoma tumours also occur; they are black in colour and spread widely in the

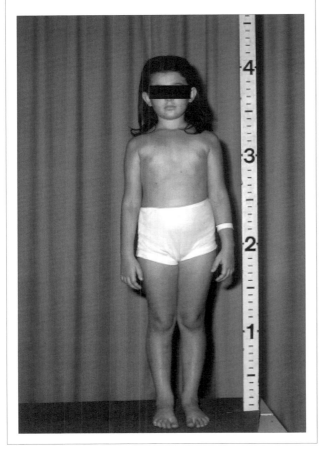

Figure 1 Female aged 7 years with an oligodendroglioma in the left parietal region of the brain which caused right facial weakness and right hemiparesis

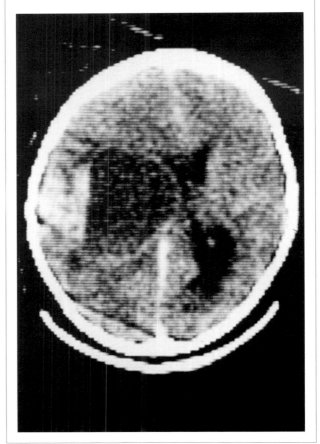

Figure 2 The oligodendroglioma in the left parietal region of the brain shown in the EMI brain scan with a cyst medial to it. The whole complex extends from the convexity almost to the midline

subarachnoid space. Although sarcoma metastases do occur, they are unusual and are very vascular and grow rapidly.

Case record A female aged 7 years was referred from another country with this history. She had been well until 2 months earlier when she had developed pain in the back of her neck and after swimming she had experienced headache; it had been noticed that her head had fallen over to the right side. She had been seen by her doctor and given medicine; she seemed to have recovered but 17 days later these symptoms had recurred following swimming. Seventeen days before consultation it had been noticed that her right arm was paralysed; one day later her right leg was also paralysed. The patient was admitted to hospital where a brain tumour was diagnosed.

During her mother's first pregnancy she had had a miscarriage at $3\frac{1}{2}$ months. This patient had had a normal birth but during this pregnancy her mother had spent much time in bed to prevent a miscarriage and had taken hydroprogesterone and allyloestrenol during the first 4 months. Her mother was aged 32 and her father aged 40 years. The child had always been healthy.

On examination she was well-built and well-nourished, intelligent and cooperative (Figure 1). Right facial weakness was noted. There were no abnormalities in the left upper extremity. In the right, there was marked weakness and diminution of voluntary movements; reflexes were brisk. There was diminished sensation in the forearm and hand. There was no muscle wasting. There was some loss of hand function on the right and some spasticity. In the lower extremities, there was no abnormality on the left. There was some function still present in the right leg but she had difficulty in walking. There was no muscle wasting. There was no patellar clonus but some ankle clonus, and knee and ankle reflexes were brisk and the plantar response was extensor. There was no obvious loss of sensation.

The patient was admitted to hospital and fully investigated. A tumour of the left parietal lobe of the brain was diagnosed. An EMI scan showed a large intracerebral tumour in the left parietal region, with a cyst medial to it. The whole complex of the tumour and the cyst extended from the convexity almost to the midline (Figure 2).

At operation, the neurosurgeon found a large well-demarcated tumour which was removed totally, except for small tumour fringes medially which were attached to the ventricular ependyma and the over-lying branches of the displaced anterior cerebral artery. The white matter surrounding the tumour was of a tougher consistency than normal and therefore might well have been involved by tumour. Histopathology appearances were those of an oligodendroglioma with scanty mitoses.

The patient showed an excellent recovery from her hemiparesis, the only residua evident being in the lack of skilled movements in her right hand. She was alert and oriented and was beginning to use her right hand for feeding purposes; she was encouraged to use chalks and crayons. A course of postoperative radiotherapy was given to the lateral and anterior left skull, with a tumour dose of 4260 R. The patient returned to her own country nearly 2 months after her first visit; physiotherapy and exercises were to continue.

The patient returned for assessment after 6 months. She walked well and had no weakness. Upper limb movements were normal except for finer movements; in the lower limbs, movements were full and normal. Clinically the central nervous system seemed normal. The EMI scan showed an appearance that might have been caused by recurrent tumour, but one could not be sure that this was not due to the operation and postoperative radiotherapy. It was decided to give no further treatment at that time as the patient was well and asymptomatic.

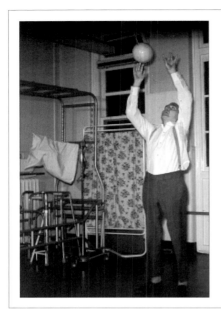

Figure 3 Patient with right hemiplegia caused by a hypernephroma metastasis in the left parietal lobe, fully rehabilitated

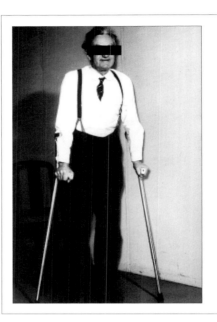

Figure 4 Male patient with a lymphoma causing compression of the spinal cord at the 6th segment, with paraplegia below this level and severe pain. He was treated with a full course of radiotherapy to the tumour and complete regression occurred. Rehabilitation restored full ambulation; this illustration shows the patient ambulant using elbow supports

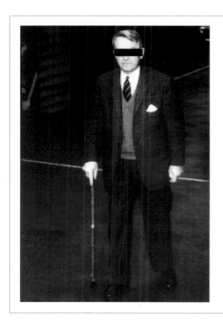

Figure 5 The same patient completely rehabilitated and walking to work

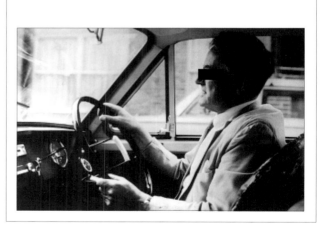

Figure 6 The same patient, resettled at work, is seen driving his motor car with modifications for a disabled driver

When reviewed after a further 3 months, the patient looked well; recently she had had two attacks of numbness in the right hand; she was able to move the right upper extremity satisfactorily and had no difficulty in walking. An EMI scan showed complete loss of the central portion of the cerebral tumour, which was replaced by a massive cyst; the walls of the cyst were lined by tumour mass.

A left parietal craniotomy was performed to remove the recurrent tumour which was dissected from the underlying white matter so that the entire cyst wall was removed. Histopathology showed that the cyst wall was composed of atypical cells bearing some resemblance to the original tumour but showing mitoses. Presumably the character of the tumour had been changed by radiotherapy, as it seemed more invasive.

The patient made a good recovery from the operation. A course of chemotherapy with N,N-bis (2-chloroethyl)-N-nitrosourea (BCNU) followed by methyl N-(2-chloroethyl)-N^1-cyclohexyl-N-nitrosourea (CCNU) was given and she returned on this treatment to her country.

She returned for review after 3 months. She was going to school daily. The upper and lower extremities appeared normal and she walked well.

The EMI scan showed recurrence of the brain tumour with finger-like processes extending deeply. No further surgical treatment was advised and a decision was made to give combined radiotherapy and chemotherapy with the objective of keeping this tumour clinically quiescent for as long as possible. A course of radiotherapy was given to the left lateral skull area, with a tumour dose of 2130 R. Chemotherapy with BCNU and vincristine was also given. She returned to her country to continue chemotherapy with methyl CCNU every 6 weeks; she was also treated with dexamethasone 0.5 mg b.d. and epinutine 50 mg h.s.

The patient returned for review 8 months later. She had recently developed numbness in the right hand and foot and some dysphasia. Examination showed full movements in the right upper and lower extremities; reflexes were a little increased. It was advised that she continue the same treatment.

An EMI scan showed further enlargement of the tumour which was extensively infiltrating the brain but producing little displacement of the ventricular system. Further surgery was considered inadvisable and the patient was to continue with dexamethasone and anticonvulsants as before.

One year and 8 months later it was reported that she had a left hemiplegia and her condition had seriously deteriorated and she had lost her eyesight. No further reports about this patient were received.

Hypernephroma metastasis in the brain
The case of a male patient with a right hemiplegia caused by a hypernephroma metastasis in the left parietal lobe which was treated with radiotherapy is illustrated in Figure 3.

THE SPINAL CORD

The different segments of the spinal cord can be affected and compressed by various tumours causing severe paralyses. Thus a chordoma of the nasopharynx can compress the cervical segment of the spinal cord and cause tetraplegia, as described in Chapter 4.

Figures 4–6 illustrate the case of a male patient with a lymphoma which caused pressure on the 6th dorsal segment of the spinal cord and paraplegia below this level. In addition to the serious paralysis, he experienced severe pain. The lymphoma was treated with a full course of radiotherapy and this successfully controlled the tumour, thus relieving the cord compression. He was rehabilitated and became fully ambulant and enabled to drive a disabled person's

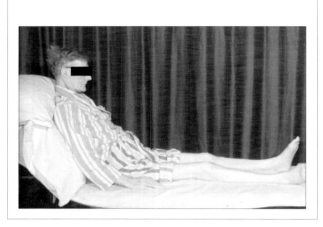

Figure 7 Male patient with a lesion of the cauda equina caused by a local recurrent carcinoma of the rectum after an abdominoperineal resection of the rectum. The recurrent carcinoma regressed with a course of radiotherapy. The patient with a flaccid paralysis of the lower extremities was rehabilitated and walked well

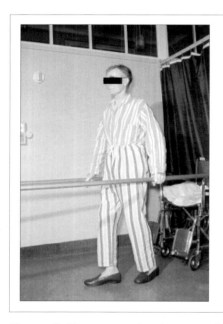

Figure 8 The same patient is seen walking between bars

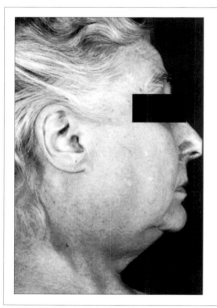

Figure 9 Female aged 61 years with a neurilemmoma in the right side of her neck causing a swelling in the right parotid salivary gland region extending into the anterior triangle of the neck

motor car. He was successfully resettled at his work as a school teacher.

CAUDA EQUINA

The cauda equina includes all the spinal nerve roots below the 2nd lumbar nerve roots; thus, the motor and sensory symptoms resulting from compression of this structure depend upon the particular roots involved. The motor symptoms are of the lower motor neuron type with flaccid paralysis and muscle atrophy. There is sensory loss over the area supplied by the four lower lumbar and all the sacral dorsal nerve roots.

Cauda equina lesions are caused by spreading primary carcinoma in the pelvic organs and also by recurrent tumours there. These lesions cause considerable pelvic pain and various degrees of incapacity.

Figures 7 and 8 illustrate the case of a patient with a cauda equina lesion caused by recurrent carcinoma of the rectum following an abdominoperineal excision for a primary carcinoma. He developed a flaccid paralysis of the lower extremities. His carcinoma was treated with a course of radiotherapy and tumour regression occurred. The patient was rehabilitated and enabled to walk well.

Neurilemmoma

A neurilemmoma is seldom found inside the skull except as a solitary tumour of the auditory (8th) cranial nerve; in that location it becomes large and compresses the pons, medulla oblongata and the cerebellum. The tumour is encapsulated and does not invade the brain or spinal cord. It is usually round and nodular with a glistening surface, hard in consistency and white or orange-white in colour. Sometimes cysts are present in the tumour, as evidence of old haemorrhage. In the spinal canal these tumours usually occur on the posterior nerve roots, either within or outside the dura mater. Occasionally they extend

through an intervertebral foramen into the thoracic or abdominal cavity. A neurilemmoma sometimes develops in the neck or in the distal portions of the upper and lower extremities.

There are two different arrangements in the histopathological structure of the tumour. One arrangement consists of cells forming interlacing bundles running in various directions. The cells have elongated nuclei which frequently grow in parallel rows. In the other arrangement, the cells are loose and reticulated; cysts of various sizes are often present. Some cells show fatty degeneration.

Case record A female aged 61 years had noticed a swelling in the right side of her neck 5 years earlier, and this had gradually increased in size. There was no pain. On examination, an oval swelling was found, 10 cm long and firm in consistency, in the region of the right parotid salivary gland and extending into the anterior triangle of the neck (Figure 9). The swelling bulged into the right lateral wall of the oropharynx and the carotid blood vessels were displaced anteriorly. There was no paralysis of nerves and no enlarged lymph nodes.

At operation, a right submandibular incision was made which extended from the mastoid process to the submental region. The sternomastoid muscle was displaced and the tumour, which was partly cystic and partly solid, was identified; it displaced the carotid blood vessels anteriorly. The vagus nerve was stretched over its external surface and the spinal accessory nerve was in contact with its superior pole. The tumour was easily dissected from the surrounding tissues and completely removed. The patient made a good recovery (Figure 10). Figure 11 shows the histopathology of the tumour.

Case record A female aged 58 years gave the history of a lump in the right side of her neck which had been present for 2 years. She had experienced recurrent attacks of tonsillitis. On examination, a tumour was

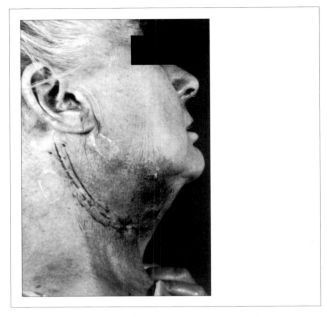

Figure 10 The neurilemmoma was excised through a submandibular incision; the healed neck after the operation

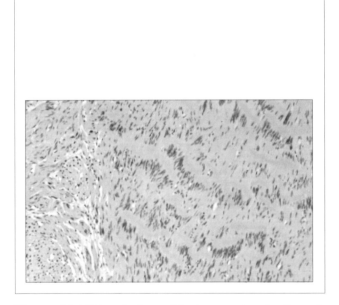

Figure 11 Histopathology of the tumour showing the cells forming interlacing bundles; the nuclei are delicate and elongated and growing in parallel rows – palisading of the nuclei

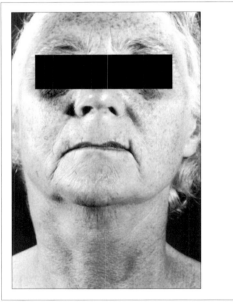

Figure 12 Female aged 58 years with a neurilemmoma of the right vagus nerve which was excised. The tumour caused a swelling in the upper third of her neck deep to the sternomastoid muscle

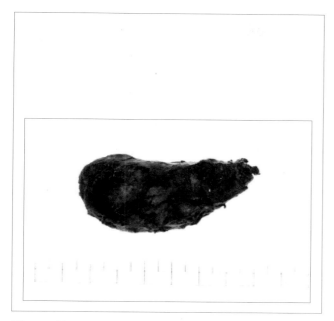

Figure 13 The excised tumour, 4 × 2 cm, was pinky-yellow in colour and it was necessary to excise a segment of the vagus nerve with the tumour

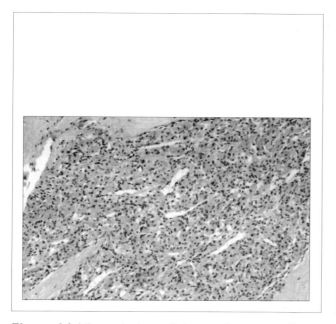

Figure 14 Histopathology of the neurilemmoma (Figure 12) showing the typical appearance

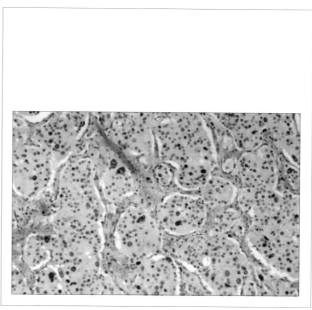

Figure 15 Histopathology of the excised segment of the vagus nerve (Figure 12)

found in the upper third of the right side of her neck deep to the sternomastoid muscle, measuring 4 × 2 cm (Figure 12). The patient coughed when the tumour was palpated.

At operation, the right side of her neck was explored and a tumour was found in continuity with the right vagus nerve. During excision the patient coughed. The tumour was pinky-yellow in colour and it was necessary to remove a segment of the right vagus nerve with the tumour (Figure 13). The patient made a good recovery from this operation; there was some voice weakness but no other ill-effects and there was no recurrence of the tumour, which was a neurilemmoma (Figures 14 and 15).

16

Tumours of the skin

Tumours both innocent and malignant often affect the skin, and this is not surprising when we consider this large expanse of tissue which is exposed to many carcinogenic agents. Some malignant tumours are more common than others, but many are now diagnosed at a much earlier stage today than formerly, and we now recognize the causes of skin tumours and thus are able to prevent their occurrence. Excessive exposure to sunlight can induce malignant melanoma of the skin and this tumour shows an increased incidence. The risk of skin cancer developing from exposure to X-radiation in the pioneer radiologists and radiographers was soon recognized and effective methods of protection were introduced, so that this form of skin cancer is rarely seen today.

The fundamental observation by Pervicall Pott in 1775 that cancer of the skin of the scrotum is common in chimney sweepers, due to the lodgement of soot in the rugae of the scrotal skin, attracted considerable professional interest and in retrospect we can recognize his work as the first step in the scientific study of chemical carcinogenesis.

The important subject of occupational skin cancer was discussed in detail by Ingram and Comaish[1]. They called attention to the large number of cases of skin cancer recorded in England which were caused chiefly by contact with coal soot, tar pitch, creosote, anthracene oils, wax and arsenicals. These authors stated that the effects of arsenic are seen in metal workers and smelters, handlers of insecticides and sheep dip and in vineyard workers. They considered that this danger arises more from inhalation and ingestion than from skin contact. They called attention to the fact that Jonathan Hutchinson was the first to describe the carcinogenic effects of the treatment of psoriasis with arsenic in the year 1887.

Figures 1 and 2 are examples of occupational skin cancers.

MOLLUSCUM SEBACEUM – KERATO ACANTHOMA

This is a benign lesion of the skin which, according to Ingram[2], was once diagnosed and treated as an acute epithelium because its clinical and histopathology appearances suggested that diagnosis. In the short period of a few weeks a small tumour with a central horny area and a fleshy base arises and suggests an acute malignant lesion (Figure 3). The tumour may be reddish in colour which, according to Ingram, suggests an inflamed sebaceous cyst. He stated that these lesions are common in pitch and tar workers and usually occur in exposed skin. They may reach up to 2.5 cm in diameter and depth and disappear spontaneously, usually in 4–6 months if left alone, leaving a depressed scar.

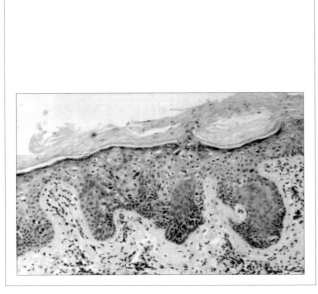

Figure 1 Skin: arsenical keratosis and carcinoma *in situ*. Histopathology appearance showing the marked cellular irregularity

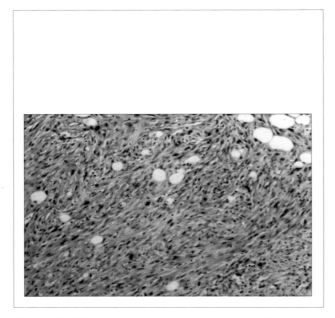

Figure 2 Skin: radiation-induced carcinoma. Histopathology appearance

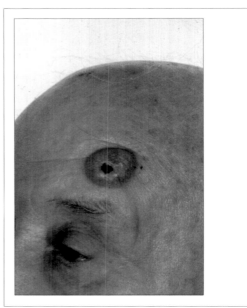

Figure 3 Molluscum sebaceum of the skin of the left frontal region

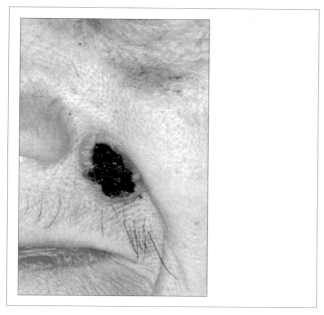

Figure 4 Basal cell carcinoma of the skin of the left cheek

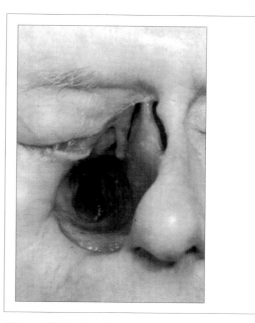

Figure 5 Basal cell carcinoma of the skin of the right face involving the inner canthus of the eye and the side of the nose

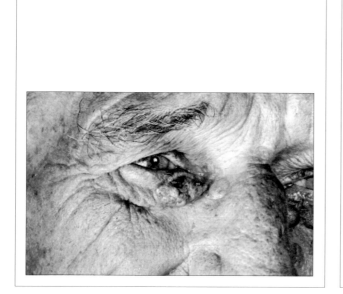

Figure 6 Basal cell carcinoma of the right lower eyelid

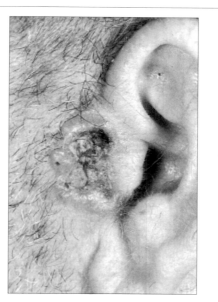

Figure 7 Basal cell carcinoma of the skin of the left pre-auricular region

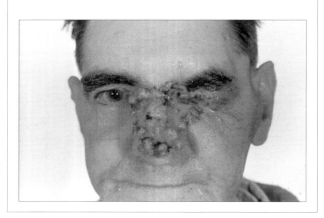

Figure 8 Basal cell carcinoma in a male patient, affecting the skin of the entire nose, left inner canthus involving the upper and lower eyelids, and the inner canthus of the right eye

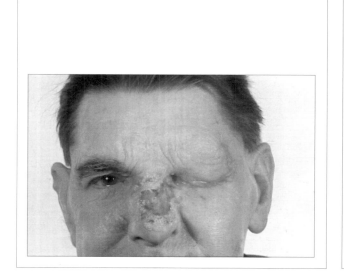

Figure 9 The same tumour showing marked regression and healing following high-voltage radiotherapy

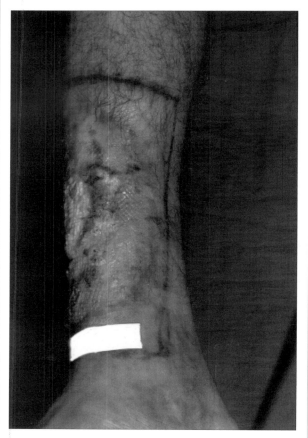

Figure 10 Squamous cell carcinoma of the skin of the leg in a male patient. This extensive carcinoma was not controlled by radiotherapy so a below-knee amputation was performed

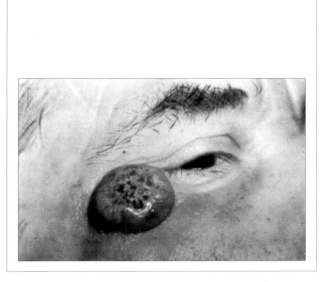

Figure 11 Squamous cell carcinoma of the skin of the outer side of the right orbit before treatment

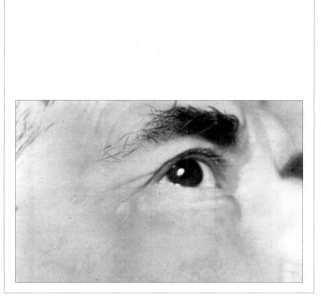

Figure 12 The same tumour after treatment with radiotherapy showing the good cosmetic result

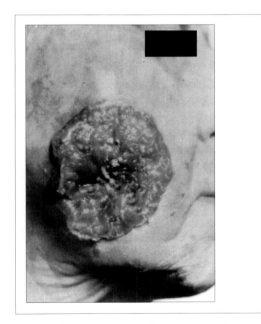

Figure 13 Squamous cell carcinoma of the skin of the right cheek before treatment

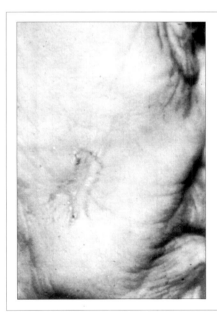

Figure 14 The same large tumour showing the good cosmetic result after radiotherapy

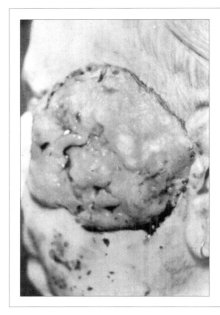

Figure 15 Squamous cell carcinoma of the skin in the upper part of the face, pre-auricular and left temple regions

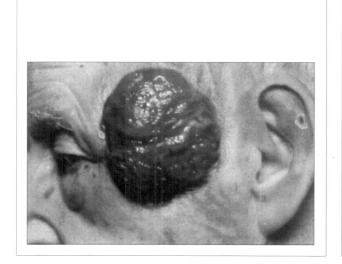

Figure 16 Squamous cell carcinoma, anaplastic variety, in the upper face and left temple region

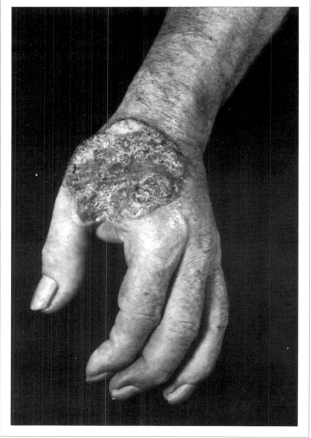

Figure 17 Squamous cell carcinoma of the skin of the hand

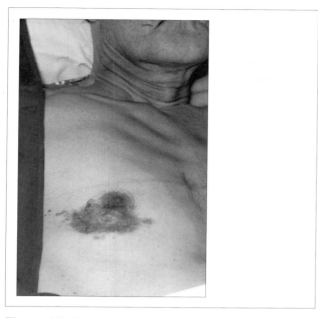

Figure 18 Skin metastasis in the chest wall from an oat cell carcinoma of the lung in a male patient

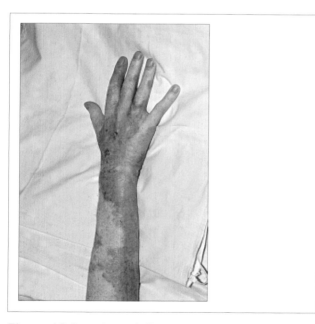

Figure 19 Lymphoma infiltration of the skin of the hand

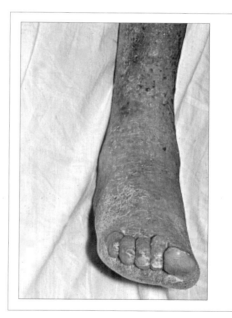

Figure 20 Lymphoma infiltration of the skin of the leg

BASAL CELL CARCINOMA (RODENT ULCER)

This malignant tumour of the skin may occur in any site but is usually seen in the skin of the face of patients in the middle and later age groups. These are locally destructive tumours and can invade adjacent bone, but they do not form metastases and they grow slowly. The tumour may be raised and hypertrophic or ulcerating with a raised rolled edge.

The diagnosis is usually made early today, so that the large tumours which are illustrated in Figures 4–7 are rare.

The usual treatment for a basal cell carcinoma is radiotherapy, when good healing will occur. A small tumour can be excised.

A male patient was referred with a very extensive and destructive basal cell carcinoma of the skin of the entire nose, left inner canthus involving the upper and lower eyelids and the inner canthus of the right eye. This tumour was treated by radiotherapy with complete regression and good healing (Figures 8 and 9).

SQUAMOUS CELL CARCINOMA

Squamous cell carcinoma of the skin is less common than basal cell carcinoma. This tumour spreads somewhat slowly to deep tissues and metastases develop in the regional lymph nodes from large tumours, but haematogenous dissemination is rarely seen. These tumours are diagnosed today usually in an early stage of development, so that extensive squamous cell carcinomas of the skin are becoming somewhat rare. The illustrations of patients treated many years ago are therefore of interest.

Regarding treatment of these tumours, if the tumour is small, complete surgical excision can be performed; larger tumours often respond favourably to a full course of radiotherapy. Metastatic regional lymph nodes should be excised if possible.

A male patient had a very extensive squamous cell carcinoma of the skin of the leg (Figure 10) which was not controlled by radiotherapy, so a below-knee amputation of the leg was performed; he was fitted with a prosthesis and was able to dress normally, and he returned to his work in another country.

A squamous cell carcinoma may occur in the skin of the face where surgical excision would be very difficult, and it is fortunate that complete regression can occur in the tumour following radiotherapy with a good cosmetic result as shown in Figures 11–14.

Figures 15–17 show large squamous cell carcinomas which are rare today.

CARCINOMA METASTASES IN THE SKIN

The skin is a fairly common site for metastases from carcinoma of certain primary tumours, as in the breast. It is rare to see a skin metastasis from an oat cell carcinoma of the lung as illustrated in Figure 18.

LYMPHOMA OF THE SKIN

A patient with lymphoma may have deposits infiltrating the skin. Figures 19 and 20 are of a patient who had deposits of lymphoma in the skin of the hand and leg. The treatment in such a case is the general management of this disease, including chemotherapy.

REFERENCES

1. Ingram, J. T. and Comaish, S. (1967). Occupational cancer of the skin. In Raven, R. W. and Rose, F. J. C. (eds.) *The Prevention of Cancer,* pp. 216–25. (London: Butterworth and Co.)
2. Ingram, J. T. (1958). Malignant tumours of the skin. In Raven, R. W. (ed.) *Cancer,* Vol. 4, Ch. 26. (London: Butterworth and Co.)

17

Tumours of bone

Tumours of bone, both the benign and malignant varieties, form a very diverse group and are divided into a number of subgroups. In this chapter the bone tumours of which the author has personal experience are described. Primary malignant tumours of bone are not common, whereas metastatic tumours are seen much more frequently. Carcinoma of the breast and prostate are well known primary tumours which metastasize to the skeleton.

BENIGN TUMOURS

Fibroma
Occasionally this tumour arises in connection with the jaws. It usually originates in the periosteum and often contains spicules of bone. It occurs in the alveolar margin of the mandible and is known as a fibrous epulis.

Myxoma
This is a rare tumour of bone and it develops in the medullary cavity, where it may become large.

Chondroma
This is a more common benign tumour arising from the epiphyseal line of a bone, and it is composed of hyaline cartilage. Common sites are the small bones of the hands and feet, and the tumours are frequently multiple. They are rounded and hard and may be become quite large. They are enclosed in connective tissue. They cause considerable deformity and may interfere with the function of joints.

Figures 1–5 show the radiological appearances of a patient with multiple chondromas.

CHONDROSARCOMA

A chondrosarcoma is a malignant tumour that arises from cartilage or connective tissue; the designation is applied solely to purely cartilaginous tumours, and they vary considerably in malignant potential. Some chondrosarcomas have their origin in a pre-existing chondroma and others arise *de novo*. They are more common in males than in females and are usually found affecting the pelvic bones and the long bones such as the humerus and femur.

Appearance
When the tumour is well-differentiated and slow-growing, the tissue resembles normal cartilage. It is bluish-white and translucent with a lobulated surface. There may be areas of calcification and bone replacement, and areas of degeneration have a gelatinous appearance. The poorly-differentiated, rapidly-growing tumour resembles less normal cartilage and may have a gelatinous or mucoid appearance. The tumour may occur centrally or in the periphery of the bone.

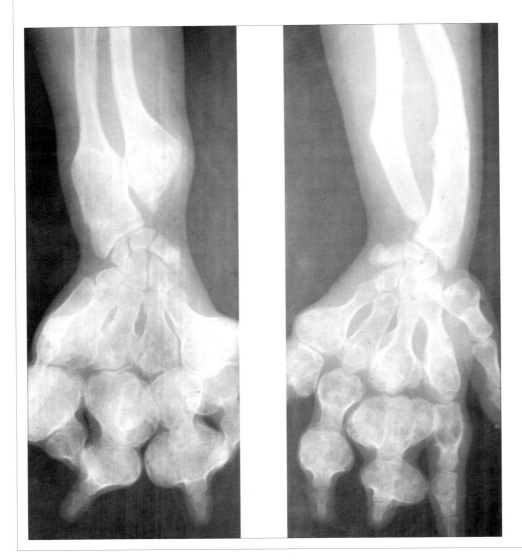

Figure 1 Radiograph of a patient with multiple chondromas of the hands causing severe deformity and dysfunction

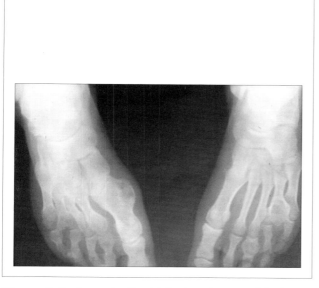

Figure 2 Radiograph of multiple chondromas of the bones of the feet

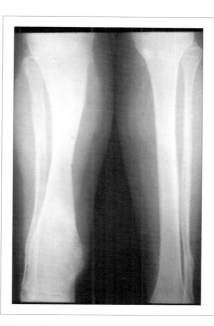

Figure 3 Radiograph of the same patient showing a chondroma of the right tibia

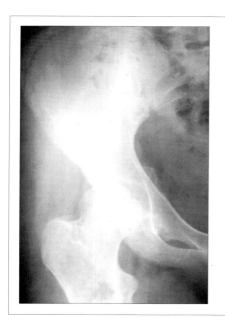

Figure 4 Multiple chondromas in the upper end of the femur involving the hip joint

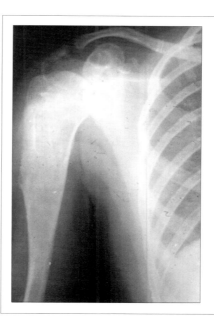

Figure 5 The same patient showing tumours in the upper part of the humerus and shoulder joint

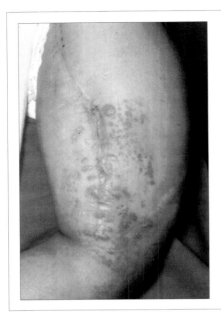

Figure 6 Female aged 25 years with recurrent tumours of the left humerus excised in another country; she had a swollen and painful left arm and a large tumour involving the upper half of the left humerus with a pathological fracture; the appearances were of a chondrosarcoma

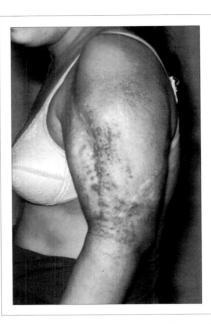

Figure 7 Diminution of the swelling of the left arm following a course of radiotherapy. The patient retained satisfactory function of the forearm, hand and fingers and continued her work as a secretary

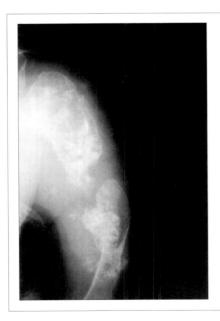

Figure 8 Radiogram of the same patient showing a huge tumour of the left humerus extending into the head, which is subluxated downwards and outwards; a pathological fracture is present and there are areas of calcification in the soft tissues

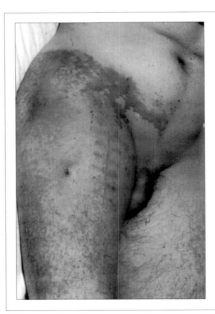

Figure 9 Male aged 36 years with a chondrosarcoma of the right femur

Histopathology

The histopathology of a slow-growing chondrosarcoma resembles that of a benign chondroma. There are areas of well-differentiated tumour cartilage, consisting of small round cells separated by abundant intercellular matrix and very few blood vessels. The rapidly-growing tumour consists of highly cellular less differentiated cartilaginous tissue which is more vascular. Chondroid intercellular matrix may be absent in parts of the tumour; collagenous or mucoid intercellular material may be present where the cells are spindle-shaped.

Spread of the tumour

Chondrosarcoma spreads locally by direct extension into contiguous tissues, so that recurrence following resection may occur. Metastases are unusual in the regional lymph nodes. The usual method of spread is by the bloodstream to form metastases in the lungs and in other organs.

Case record   A female aged 25 years was referred with this history. Ten years previously a tumour of the left arm had been excised in another country. Two years later another tumour of the left arm had been excised and 18 months following this operation a third tumour of the left arm had been excised. No histopathology of these tumours was available.

The patient presented with a tumour of the left humerus present for 1 year. Examination showed a swollen, painful and tender left shoulder with a plaster in position, and scars of previous operations (Figure 6). In the right lower extremity there was a hard, fixed tumour 15 × 10 cm in the right femur.

It is interesting that this patient's father, sister and brother had had tumours excised from the lower limbs and the patient was a known case of 'multiple exostosis in a diaphyseal aclasis' syndrome.

X-ray examination showed a pathological fracture through the upper humerus, which was the site of a large bone tumour. There was also evidence of diaphyseal aclasis in the right humerus and forearm. In the lower limbs, changes of diaphyseal aclasis were present in both limbs. The radiological appearances of the upper half of the shaft of the left humerus showed that the chondromas had become sarcomatous, with a fracture through the sarcomatous area.

The patient did not wish to have a dislocation amputation through the left shoulder joint. The metal rod splinting the fracture was therefore removed and multiple biopsies were taken, but the histopathology was non-specific of a tumour. A course of radiotherapy was given to the tumour of the upper left humerus with a dose of 6000 R. The left arm improved and was less swollen and the function of the left upper extremity was much better (Figure 7); the patient was satisfied with this useful limb. The patient returned to her own country.

The patient was examined 3 months later and she stated that she was able to use her left upper extremity and type as a secretary. There was a large tumour of the upper left humerus projecting into the axilla, and a false joint in the mid-humerus. A radiograph showed a huge tumour involving the upper three-quarters of the humerus extending into the head, which was subluxated downwards and outwards; irregular calcification was evident in the tumour and soft tissues and an ununited fracture was present (Figure 8). There were no metastases in the lungs or bony thorax.

A biopsy operation on the tumour was carried out with the following histopathology. The biopsies consisted almost entirely of very cellular cartilage with only a few foci of calcification. There was considerable variation in the size and shape of the nuclei and multinucleate cells were fairly frequent. No mitotic figures were seen but the histological appearances were considered to be those of a low-grade well-differentiated chondrosarcoma.

Further treatment was carefully considered and discussed with the patient who stated that she would not have any amputation of the left upper extremity. This decision was accepted since the patient had good function of the forearm, hand and fingers enabling her to work as a secretary, and the tumour was of low malignancy. A further course of radiotherapy was given to the left humerus. Her general condition was very satisfactory; there was no evidence of metastases and she had very little pain. The patient returned to her own country finally 3 years and 7 months after her first visit. No further follow-up information was received.

This case has many interesting features. The patient had the diaphyseal aclasis syndrome which seems to have been familial in her father, sister and brother. Over a period of several years, recurrent tumours were excised from her left arm. She developed a chondrosarcoma of the left humerus; the treatment described enabled the patient to continue her work as a secretary over several years. No metastases were demonstrated during the follow-up period.

Case record A male aged 36 years was referred from another country with the history of having developed pain in his right knee 3 years previously; pain had occurred in the right groin 9 months before the consultation. A swelling had appeared in the right thigh 3 months earlier and this had been explored and biopsied by a surgeon in his country. Histopathology showed a chondrosarcoma.

On examination, there was a healed scar in the right thigh and an ill-defined swelling 15 × 10 cm, which was firm and fixed (Figure 9). Radiograms of the right thigh and pelvis showed a large soft tissue mass on the medial aspect of the upper part of the right thigh. Associated with this there was destruction of the lesser trochanter of the femur and an irregular area of cortical bone lying adjacent. No abnormality was noted in the hip joint or pelvic bones. The appearances were those of a malignant tumour in the upper part of the right thigh, which was mostly in the soft tissues but was destroying the lesser trochanter. No metastases were seen on chest X-ray.

A preoperative course of radiotherapy was administered to the right thigh and lower right pelvis, with a total dose of 4948 R. One month later the right groin was surgically explored and the external iliac lymph nodes were excised; frozen section histopathology showed no tumour. The right lower extremity was then amputated by disarticulation at the hip joint. The patient made a good recovery from this operation.

Histopathology sections from the right femur and the soft tissue mass showed moderately differentiated chondrosarcoma. The tissue was cellular and there were numerous plump nuclei and binucleate forms. In one block the bone and tumour tissue showed necrosis, but the tumour tissue in other blocks was viable and active. A femoral node and external iliac nodes showed no evidence of tumour.

The patient was fitted with a tilting-table limb prosthesis and was rehabilitated; he walked well and his general condition was satisfactory. He returned to his own country. Seven months after his amputation he was reportedly very mobile and was taking short walks. He was followed up in his own country and no further details were made available.

OSTEOSARCOMA

An osteosarcoma is a very lethal tumour which arises from the skeletal connective tissue and usually shows the formation of osteoid or bony intercellular matrix. The tumour may arise in bones affected by Paget's disease. The long bones are usually affected, especially towards the end of the shafts, but an osteosarcoma can affect any part of the skeleton. Occasionally this tumour is radiation-induced and can follow irradiation of a benign tumour of bone (see Figure 10).

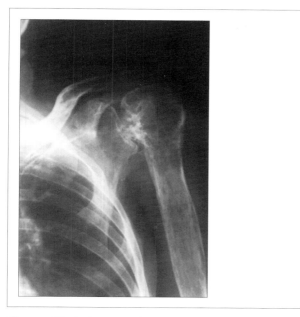

Figure 10 Radiogram of a radiation-induced osteosarcoma of the upper end of the humerus

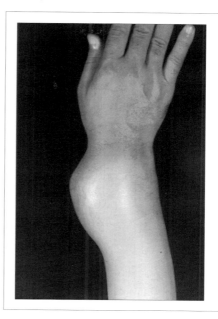

Figure 11 Male aged 30 years with an osteosarcoma of the lower end of the right radius

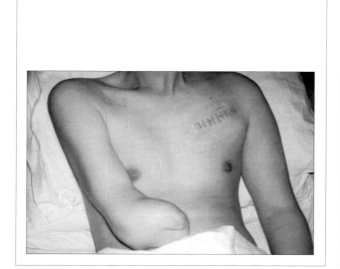

Figure 12 The amputation stump following below-elbow amputation of the right upper extremity

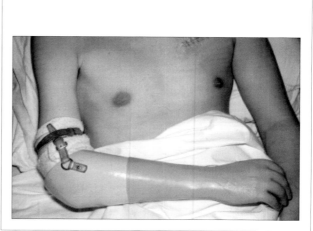

Figure 13 The same patient wearing his arm prosthesis; he acquired full movement of his right elbow joint

Appearance

An osteosarcoma usually arises centrally in the bone and causes it to expand. The cut surface of the tumour may show areas of bone which are sometimes interspersed with vascular non-ossified areas and necrotic tissue. The bone cortex is eroded and the periosteum displaced. The soft tissues around the tumour are invaded and a pathological fracture may occur following bone destruction. A considerable degree of ossification in the tumour is often seen.

Histopathology

The appearances are variable in different tumours but generally the tumour cells are similar to osteoblasts. Areas of anaplastic undifferentiated spindle cell tissue showing mitoses are usually present, and varying amounts of bony differentiation with the formation of osteoid or bony matrix by tumour cells are seen.

Methods of spread

Osteosarcoma spreads within the bone from the centre to the periosteum and into the contiguous soft tissues. Metastases in the regional lymph nodes are rare. The chief method of spread is by the bloodstream, which occurs early in the disease. Metastases are formed in the lungs and in other organs and tissues.

Case record A male aged 30 years gave the history of a tumour in the right lower radius increasing in size over more than 1 year. Examination showed a large tumour arising from the lower third of the right radius, elastic in consistency; the skin over it was hotter than its surroundings (Figure 11). Movements at the right wrist joint, especially flexion, were limited. The regional lymph nodes were not enlarged.

A radiogram showed expansion and destruction of the lower end of the right radius. Associated with this there was a large soft tissue mass and there was a considerable amount of bone formation extending into the mass. No lung metastases were present.

A biopsy was performed for histopathology. The specimens were described as several irregular portions of pinkish-grey soft tissue and tiny bone fragments, which were portions of an osteosarcoma displaying much tumour osteoid and bone formation. Nuclear pleomorphism and hyperchromasia were prominent features. There was moderate mitotic activity.

An amputation of the right upper extremity below the elbow joint was performed. The patient made a good recovery from this operation and was fitted with a right arm prosthesis; he achieved a full range of movement at the right elbow joint (Figures 12 and 13). Three years and 3 months later the patient returned from his own country with a large metastasis in the left upper chest involving the upper lobe of the lung. A biopsy for histopathology was reported as fragments of malignant tumour with a distinct osteogenic pattern: metastatic osteosarcoma. The patient returned to his own country and was lost to follow-up.

Figure 14 shows an osteosarcoma of the tibia with ulceration of the overlying skin.

RETICULUM CELL SARCOMA

The distinction between the reticulum cell sarcoma and Ewing's tumour is difficult to define on the basis of their clinical features and radiological appearances. Many patients with reticulum cell sarcoma are adolescents or young adults and this tumour is more common in males than females. The tumour is usually situated in the shaft of long bones, especially the femur.

Case record A male aged 14 years gave the history of having developed pain in the left knee joint, and in another country an exploratory operation had been carried out. Tuberculosis had been diagnosed and he had received antituberculosis treatment. Later a surgical biopsy had been done and the histopathology was reported as showing a malignant synovioma. A course of radiotherapy had been given.

On examination of the left knee joint healed skin scars were found; a bony swelling affected both condyles of the femur and this was more marked in the medial condyle (Figure 15). Flexion of the joint was limited to 90° and there was a little lateral mobility. A radiogram showed gross abnormality of the lower end of the shaft of the left femur. The lower epiphysis was completely disorganized, and there was widening of the shaft affecting both condyles, with slight thickening of the cortex posteriorly (Figure 16); some of this may have been due to the previous operations. There was no evidence of disseminated disease.

The histopathology slides of the original biopsy were reviewed and the appearances were those of a highly malignant undifferentiated tumour of mesodermal origin, composed of sheets of cells with a poorly defined rim of cytoplasm and large vesicular nuclei, with prominent nucleoli. There was some dense hyaline stroma. There was no evidence of malignant synovioma or osteosarcoma. The appearances were suggestive of reticulum cell sarcoma.

A biopsy of a left cervical and left inguinal lymph node was performed and histopathology showed no abnormality. Bone marrow cytology was normal. The patient was kept under careful observation. A heavy dose of radiotherapy had already been given to the tumour with consequent regression and perhaps inactivation of the disease. There was no evidence of dissemination. A severe valgus deformity of 40° gradually developed in the left knee joint, and an orthopaedic surgeon performed a double osteotomy, lower femoral and upper tibial, to correct it. The patient made a good recovery from this operation and the bones united satisfactorily. Ultimately the left lower extremity was shortened by 10 cm and flexion

at the left knee joint was limited to 40°. The patient was able to walk well and he wore smart shoes and returned to his own country.

Nine years later the patient was well and was at work.

EWING'S TUMOUR

As already stated, the distinction between Ewing's tumour and reticulum cell sarcoma is difficult to define. Figures 17–20 are illustrations of a young adolescent male who was referred from another country with a Ewing's tumour of the right upper femur. This patient had great difficulty in walking caused by this destructive malignant tumour involving the upper shaft, neck and head of the right femur. He was treated with radiotherapy and fitted with a walking caliper, which permitted satisfactory ambulation.

SOLITARY PLASMACYTOMA OF BONE

A solitary plasmacytoma of bone is a rare tumour and this diagnosis can be accepted only if, after the onset of the supposedly solitary tumour, there is a long period of freedom from clinical and radiological evidence of myelomatosis, or if a thorough necropsy examination proves that no other tumours are present in the skeleton.

The first symptoms of a solitary plasmacytoma of bone arise in consequence of a pathological fracture caused by even a trivial injury, or pain may occur at the site of the tumour. The pain is often severe, and when the tumour is situated in the spine there may be girdle pain. Paraplegia with all its accompanying features is a serious complication caused by this tumour in the spine. Later, general symptoms occur which include weakness and secondary anaemia.

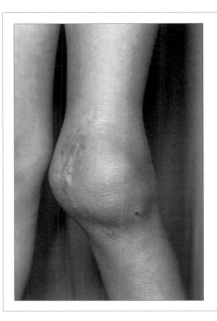

Figure 15 Male aged 14 years with a reticulum cell sarcoma of the lower end of the left femur showing healed scars from previous operations, swelling of both condyles of the femur (more marked in the medial condyle) and a valgus deformity of the knee joint. He had previously received radiotherapy

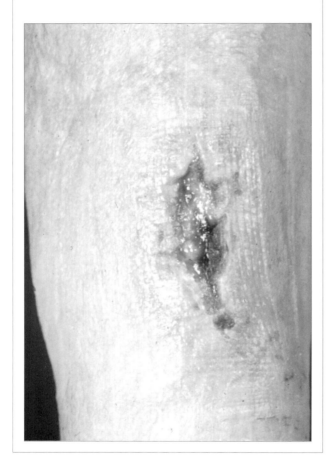

Figure 14 Patient with an osteosarcoma of the left tibia causing ulceration of the overlying skin

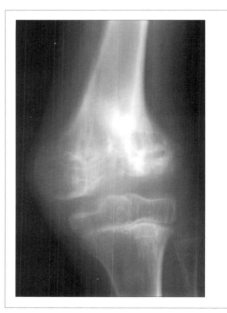

Figure 16 The radiogram shows gross abnormality of the lower end of the shaft of the femur; the lower epiphysis is completely disorganized, with widening of the shaft affecting both condyles and slight thickening of the cortex posteriorly

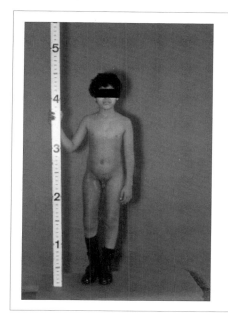

Figure 17 A young adolescent male with a Ewing's tumour of the upper shaft, neck and head of the right femur causing swelling of the right thigh and great difficulty in walking

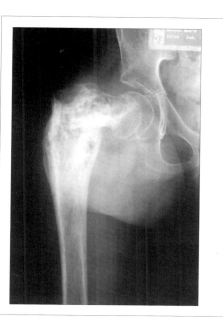

Figure 18 Radiogram showing the bone destruction of the upper femur, neck and head

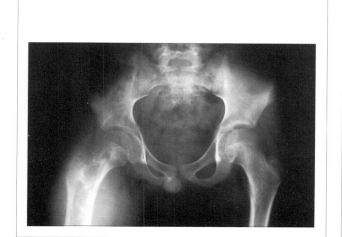

Figure 19 The radiographic appearances following radiotherapy; there is regression of the tumour and consolidation of the affected femur

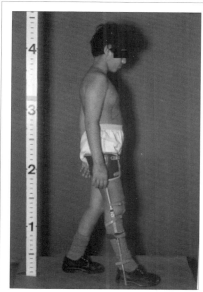

Figure 20 The patient was fitted with a walking caliper permitting satisfactory ambulation

The radiological appearances are of two main types. In one type there is a very destructive lesion involving the bone which is well demarcated and sharply defined. In some respects this resembles a carcinoma metastasis of the osteolytic variety or the osteolytic type of osteosarcoma. The other type has a cystic and trabeculated appearance, the trabeculae being thickened and irregular. The lesion is large, situated in the medulla of the bone and often expands the cortex.

Regarding treatment, these tumours are radiosensitive and following radiotherapy there may be regression and recalcification. When the tumour is situated in the spine this is the best treatment; pain is relieved even after vertebral collapse with paraplegia. If pressure paraplegia occurs, laminectomy may be required to relieve pressure on the spinal cord. There is no evidence that radiotherapy is curative. Surgical treatment has been undertaken for tumours situated in accessible sites. Thus, curettage of the tumour followed by bone grafting has been performed, and in some patients an amputation has been done.

The following case history was published by Raven and Willis[1] who also reviewed the authentic cases of this disease published in the literature.

Case record   A male aged 56 years, a tent erector, was admitted to hospital with paraplegia. Six weeks previously he had lifted a heavy weight and had felt something 'give way' in his back, and after half an hour he had experienced abdominal pain. Nine days later he had been admitted to hospital with girdle pains. At that time he noticed that his toes were numb and later they became paralysed. This paralysis extended upwards as far as the umbilicus.

On examination his general condition was good. No gross abnormality was detected in the heart and lungs and the abdomen was normal. Girdle pain and hyperaesthesia were present over the distribution of the 6th dorsal segment of the spinal cord. Below this level there was paraplegia and anaesthesia. There was incontinence of urine.

Radiograms of the spine showed forward subluxation of the 6th dorsal vertebra with incomplete destruction of two bodies, suggestive of a tumour metastasis. The rest of the spine showed no abnormality. Radiograms of the skull, pelvis, femora and humeri were normal. Urine examination showed a trace of albumin and pus cells with *Bacillus coli* and *Bacillus proteus*. Haematology was normal except for leukocytosis of 18 000 per mm^3. The erythrocyte sedimentation rate was raised at 21 mm/h (Wintrobe). Sternal marrow showed normal histopathology and no evidence of myeloma. A laminectomy was performed removing the laminae of the 6th, 7th and 8th dorsal vertebrae. A soft, friable, vascular tumour was found eroding the laminae and extending into the erector spinae muscles. The tumour surrounded the dura mater, but did not involve its posterior aspect. The spinal cord was seen to pulsate. Part of the tumour was removed for histopathology and the wound was closed. A plaster support was applied to the spine.

Histopathology showed that the tissue consisted of compact masses of characteristic plasma cells which gave a clearly defined and typical reaction with linna-Pappenheim methyl green pyronin. The tumour was identified as a plasmacytoma.

The patient's general health continued to be satisfactory for several months. The urinary bladder was drained continuously by an indwelling catheter until reflex micturition was established 6 weeks after the operation. There was complete anaesthesia with paraplegia below the 7th and 8th dorsal vertebrae and 5 weeks after the operation increasing involuntary movements developed in the legs which were partially controlled by luminal and codeine medication. The patient also complained of severe girdle pains. Five months after the operation the patient's condition deteriorated and he died 5 months and 17 days following the laminectomy operation.

At necropsy, the bodies of the 6th and 7th dorsal vertebrae were found to be completely replaced by soft, grey-pinkish tumour with collapse of the bone and free lateral mobility of the spine at this level. The intervertebral disc between the two vertebrae was largely intact and lay loosely isolated at the centre of the tumour. The tumour had spread anteriorly and laterally beneath the anterior common ligament and over the ribs and intercostal spaces for a distance of 3.5 cm on both sides of the vertebrae. It had narrowed the spinal canal and compressed the cord, but had not penetrated through the dura mater. Posteriorly there was invasion of the dorsal spinal muscles, especially on the right side. No other tumours were found after careful search in other vertebrae, sternum, skull, pelvis and shaft of the right femur; all these bones were sectioned. The shaft of the femur contained red marrow from which smears were taken. No other tumours were found elsewhere in the body.

Smears and sections of the vertebral tumour, stained with the usual haematoxylin methods and by the linna-Pappenheim method for plasma cells, showed it to be a typical plasmacytoma, with many cells of poorly differentiated, immature type, but also many well differentiated plasma cells with characteristic structure and staining properties. The cells showed a moderate number of mitotic figures. A few cells were abnormally large and contained large irregular or multiple (usually only two or three) nuclei. Stromal tissue was scanty. Small blood vessels were plentiful in some parts and there were also areas of haemorrhage and degeneration, especially in the central areas of the tumour.

Sections and smears of red marrow from other bones showed no evidence of plasma cell infiltration.

In sections of the kidney, a few tubules contained some brownish amorphous debris, probably of no special significance.

MULTIPLE MYELOMATOSIS

Multiple myelomatosis is a multifocal disease of the skeleton and especially of the bones of the trunk. It may present as a solitary lesion and later becomes widespread causing the death of the patient. The disease usually occurs in late middle life.

Symptomatology

Pain is the commonest symptom; at first it is mild but with the further development of the disease, severe paroxysms are experienced accompanying a pathological fracture of bone, which is a frequent complication. Involvement of nerve roots causes much distress. Palpable tumours are infrequent but when they occur, they are tender, small, rubbery or firm. Bone destruction with collapse of an affected vertebra can cause paraplegia. An important finding is Bence–Jones protein in the urine which occurs in about half these patients, especially in the later stages of the disease, and may be accompanied by severe renal damage.

The radiological features typically are multiple circumscribed areas of bone destruction which are small in diameter. Marrow cytology shows the typical myeloma cells.

Appearance

In diffuse myelomatosis the characteristic feature is the presence of large numbers of small nodules in the bone marrow practically confined to the sites of red marrow. They vary in colour from pale grey to a deep plum colour. The bones become thin and fragile so that a pathological fracture occurs, and extra-osseous tumours can develop which are soft and fleshy.

Histopathology

The appearances consist of a uniform sheet of my-

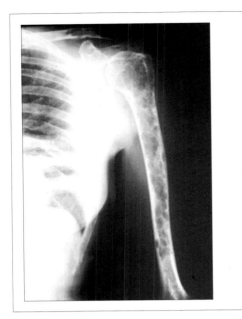

Figure 21 Female aged 41 years with multiple myelomatosis. Radiological appearances of the humerus and ribs showing multiple deposits of tumour and extensive disease. There is marked thinning of the shaft of the humerus

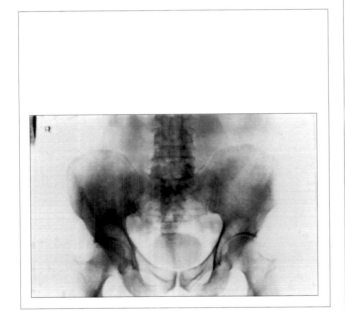

Figure 22 The radiological appearances of the multiple myelomatosis in the pelvic bones and upper ends of each femur

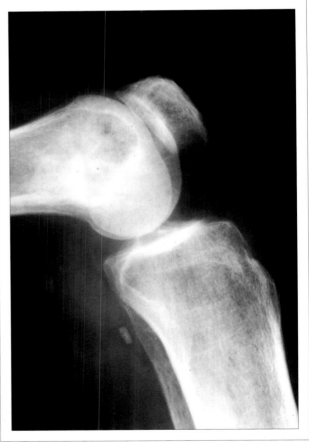

Figure 23 Patient with a carcinoma of the breast who developed metastases in her knee joint. The radiological appearances are shown here

eloma cells; large numbers are present in the red marrow and in the majority of cases they are plasma cells. Usually there is no stroma but sometimes there is a reticulum framework.

Case record　A female aged 41 years gave this history. She had developed anorexia and lassitude 15 months previously and had had vague pains in her left shoulder and chest; the pain had later extended to the spine. She had noticed some weight loss but no other symptoms.

Her general condition was fair; the conjunctivae were pale and a small mobile lymph node was present in the left posterior triangle of the neck. There was general limitation of movements in the left shoulder because of pain, and tenderness was elicited over the mid-dorsal spine.

Radiological examination showed extensive tumour deposits in the left shoulder, sternum, skull, cervical, dorsal and lumbar segments of the spine with partial collapse of most of the vertebral bodies except the upper three and the 7th dorsal vertebrae; deposits were present in the pelvic bones. Figure 21 shows the tumour deposits in the humerus and ribs. The patient received chemotherapy with some improvement except for residual sternal pain.

The patient died from a pulmonary infection 2 years and 9 months later.

As stated already, multiple myelomatosis can affect the bones of the pelvis. Figure 22 shows the radiological appearance of the pelvic bones of a patient with this disease.

CARCINOMA METASTASES IN BONE

The skeleton is a common site for carcinoma metastases from many primary sites, of which carcinoma of the breast and prostate are very common.

Figure 23 shows the radiological appearance of carcinoma metastases in the knee joint of a patient with a primary carcinoma of the breast. The knee joint is not commonly affected by metastases in this disease.

REFERENCE

1. Raven, R. W. and Willis, R. A. (1949). Solitary plasmacytoma of the spine. *J. Bone Joint Surg.*, **31B**, 369–75

18

Sarcomas of soft tissues

The majority of the sarcomas of soft tissues seem to be malignant from their onset but there are a few exceptions. For example, a large lipoma, especially in the region of the scapula, may develop into a liposarcoma; hence these large benign tumours must always be treated with careful excisional surgery. Occasionally a malignant neurilemmoma may develop in a patient with von Recklinghausen's disease, or neurofibromatosis. Soft tissue sarcomas may develop in people of all ages and they occur in infants, children and young adults.

The majority of these tumours spread by the bloodstream to form metastases in the lungs, liver and other sites. Some of them spread by the lymphatics to the regional lymph nodes; these include angiosarcoma and rhabdomyosarcoma.

FIBROSARCOMA

A fibrosarcoma may develop in any part of the body where fibrous tissue is present, and usually develops spontaneously. This tumour spreads through the bloodstream to form metastases in the liver, lungs and other sites. It may recur following excision, and metastases do occur in the regional lymph nodes.

Case record   A female aged 15 years was referred from another country with this history. At the age of

13 years the patient had fallen and fractured her right clavicle, which had been immobilized. Six months later she had fallen again and had fractured her left clavicle, which had been immobilized, and when this bandage had been removed a swelling had been found under the right clavicle (previously fractured); this had gradually increased in size. Eight months later the surgeon had examined the patient and had found a mass the size of a large orange projecting through the right infraclavicular fossa, firmly fixed to the clavicle and surrounding tissues. There were dilated veins and phlebography showed marked stenosis of the axillary vein, which was displaced downwards with reflux into the subscapular vein. There was weakness of the deltoid and brachialis anticus muscles. The surgeon operated and divided the right clavicle and removed the tumour which extended into the supraclavicular fossa; the divided clavicle was fixed with a pin, which was removed 4 weeks later.

The tumour measured 11 × 8 × 5 cm; the histopathology was reported as that of a fibroma. Nine months later the surgeon found a local recurrent tumour causing pain in the right upper extremity.

On examination a hard fixed tumour 22.5 cm long was found extending from the right clavicle into the right axilla, involving the anterior chest wall (Figure 1). The scar of the previous operation was noted; no enlarged left axillary nodes were found.

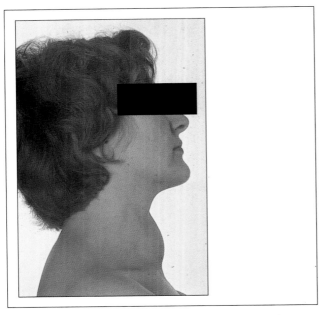

Figure 1 Female aged 15 years with a recurrent fibrosarcoma of the right upper chest wall extending beneath the clavicle into the lower neck

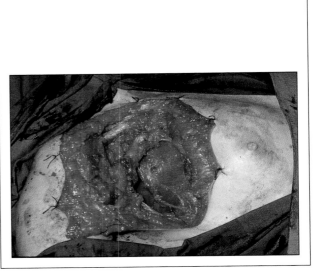

Figure 2 Surgical exposure of the tumour prior to excision

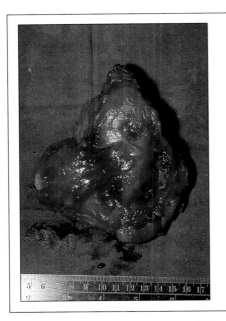

Figure 3 Operation specimen of the tumour which is imperfectly encapsulated, lobulated and infiltrating adjacent striated muscle

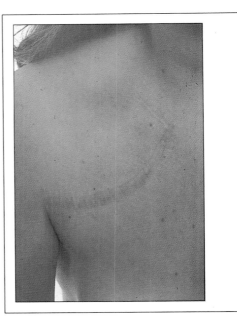

Figure 4 The healed wound after excision

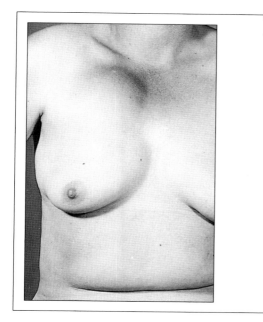

Figure 5 Female aged 45 years with a fibrosarcoma in the infraclavicular region of the right breast, 7.5 cm in diameter and fixed to the chest wall

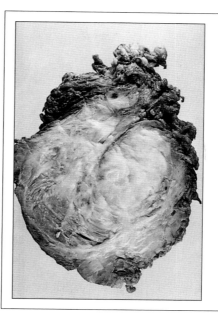

Figure 6 Specimen excised showing non-encapsulation of the tumour and the attached anterior segments of the 2nd, 3rd and 4th ribs and intervening chest wall

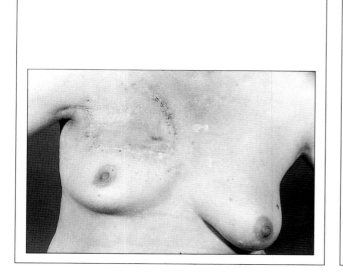

Figure 7 The healed wound following excision of the fibrosarcoma in the infraclavicular region of the right breast

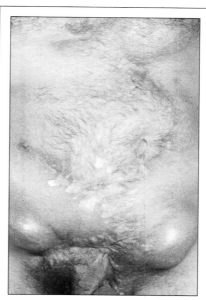

Figure 8 Male aged 29 years with recurrent fibrosarcoma of the left chest wall and both groins extending into the perineum and right side of the scrotum

Preoperative radiotherapy was administered to the whole tumour area with a total dose of 4000 R. The tumour in the right axilla was explored through the original incision with a posterior extension (Figure 2) and a large tumour was found which was difficult to remove at its upper part due to fibrosis. The lower two-thirds of the tumour was not infiltrating and was cleanly removed (Figure 3). The axillary artery, vein and nerves were stretched over the tumour, which passed behind them to the right side of the neck and deep to the clavicle. In this situation it was attached to the posterior cord of the brachial plexus which was running through the tumour and had to be resected with the tumour. The axillary vessels and nerves were conserved. The wound healed well (Figure 4). A course of postoperative radiotherapy was given.

On histopathology, the tumour was found to be a well differentiated fibrosarcoma with abundant mature collagen. The neoplasm was imperfectly encapsulated and had invaded the adjacent striated muscle in several places. A special feature was noted: in two of the lymph nodes there were crescentic collections of heavily pigmented cells at the periphery. The pigment was melanin and the cells varied from ovoid to spindle-shaped. The appearances did not suggest metastatic malignant melanoma but were similar to benign deposits of blue naevus.

This patient had had a blue naevus excised from the right little finger 5 years previously and a small pigmented spot was found in the scar; this was excised under local anaesthesia. Histopathology appearances were those of a simple blue naevus showing no features of malignancy. The pigmented deposits in the axillary lymph nodes represented benign migration of naevus cells.

Eight years following the operation a hard swelling was found in the right mid-neck, 4 cm in diameter and mobile. At surgical exploration, this cervical tumour was invading the sternomastoid muscle and extended into the lower neck, where it was fixed. As much as possible of the tumour was excised. A postoperative course of radiotherapy was given to the tumour area. Histopathology showed the tumour to be a recurrent fibrosarcoma involving the right sternomastoid muscle, relatively acellular and highly collagenized. In one or two areas the cells were slightly pleomorphic and showed a sprinkling of mitoses, but generally these were not frequent. There was no lymph node or vein involvement; one neurovascular bundle was compressed and distorted by the tumour.

Three years later following marriage the patient gave birth to a healthy daughter who was underweight. Five years after the last operation the patient sustained a fracture of the upper end of her right humerus, probably because of weakening of the bone by radiotherapy.

The patient was examined 12 years and 11 months after radiotherapy and excision of the recurrent fibrosarcoma, and no evidence of disease was found. She then left to reside in another country.

The long survival following treatment in this case is noteworthy. Of additional interest is the demonstration that a benign blue naevus can cause metastatic involvement of the regional lymph nodes.

Case record   A female aged 45 years gave the history of a swelling in the infraclavicular region of the right breast for a period of 5 years. During the previous 3 months this swelling had increased considerably in size. Examination showed a large swelling below the right clavicle 7.5 cm in diameter; it was not attached to skin, but was firmly fixed to the chest wall; it was elastic in consistency (Figure 5). Both breasts were normal. There were nodes in the axillae or neck and no evidence of metastases.

Histopathology showed a well differentiated fibrosarcoma.

Preoperative radiotherapy was given. A total excision of the tumour in the right infraclavicular region (Figure 6) was performed with the anterior segments of the 2nd, 3rd and 4th ribs and the intervening chest wall. The pleura was not opened. Figure 7 shows the healed incision.

Histopathology appearances were those of well differentiated mature fibrous tissue in which collagen formation was abundant. The cells were regular and exhibited no aberration. Mitoses were extremely rare. There was no suggestion of encapsulation and the fibrous tissue streamed out and engulfed the muscle fibres at its periphery. The histological features were those of an extra-abdominal desmoid tumour. It was thought that the behaviour of this tumour would almost certainly be similar to those growing in the abdominal wall, with a tendency to recur at long intervals, but no propensity to metastasize. The axillary lymph nodes showed reactive changes only.

The patient was examined 3 years and 11 months after her operation and no evidence of recurrence of metastases was found.

A fibrosarcoma may continue recurring following treatment over the course of many years, as exemplified by the following case.

Case record   A male aged 29 years had since the age of 9 years had recurrent tumours in the anterior abdominal wall which had been excised and had then recurred on four occasions, and radiotherapy had been given on one occasion.

Examination showed tumours in the left chest wall, and tumours in both groins fixed to the pubic bone and extending into the perineum and right side of the scrotum. There was considerable scarring at the root of the penis, and foreskin oedema (see Figure 8). All the tumours were excised and postoperative radiotherapy was given.

Histopathology showed the appearance of poorly differentiated fibrosarcoma.

Three months later the patient developed several recurrent nodules, which were excised. All the wounds healed well from these operations.

The patient returned to his own country and died 1 year and 4 months after the first of the latter two operations.

A fibrosarcoma may form metastases in the lungs (see Figure 9) from a primary tumour removed many years earlier.

ULCERATING FIBROSARCOMA

Widespread local ulceration is not common in a fibrosarcoma; a very interesting example follows of a patient who was referred from another country.

Case record   A male aged 64 years gave this history. During the previous 23 years he had had a tumour in the right iliofemoral region excised on ten occasions. It was stated that the tumour was a neurilemmoma. In addition he had had three courses of radiotherapy. During the previous 5 years there had been skin ulceration with exposure of the adjacent ilium. He had experienced increasing difficulty in walking for 1 year.

Examination showed a large tumour in the right iliofemoral region exposing the crest of the right ilium, which was black, and extending into the right anterior abdominal wall (Figure 10). Movements were painful at the right hip joint and there was difficulty in walking. Several small lymph nodes were palpable in the inguinal region. A chest radiogram showed no lung metastases. There was a defect in the right ilium.

A biopsy was done and histopathology showed a well differentiated fibrosarcoma.

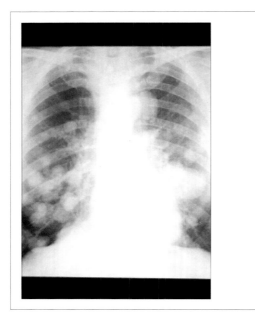

Figure 9 Male aged 57 years with metastases in the lungs from a primary fibrosarcoma of the thigh which had been excised 24 years earlier

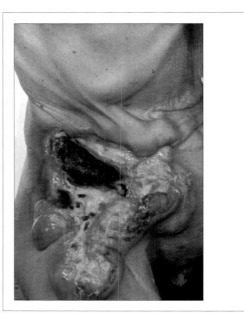

Figure 10 Male aged 64 years with an extensive fibrosarcoma in the right iliofemoral region exposing the adjacent ilium, which is black

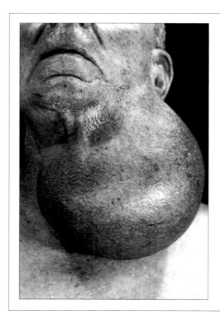

Figure 11 Male with an enormous lipoma involving the whole left side of the neck and extending upwards into the left face. This lipoma was excised

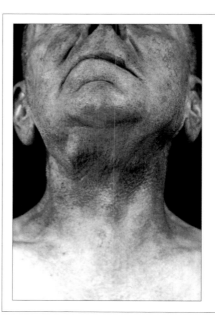

Figure 12 The good cosmetic result following surgical excision

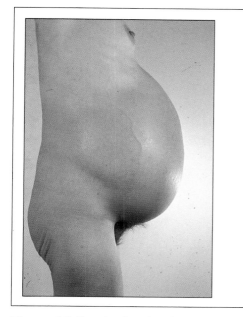

Figure 13 Female showing the swelling of the abdomen caused by a large retroperitoneal liposarcoma, which was excised

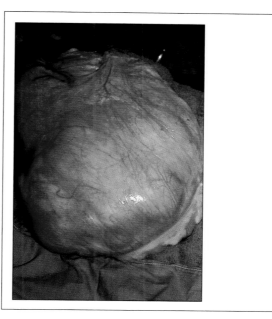

Figure 14 The specimen of the tumour showing lobulation and vascularity

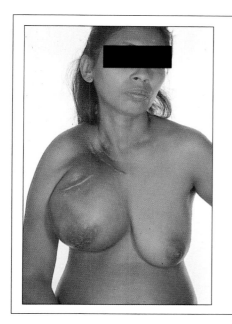

Figure 15 Female aged 55 years with a large recurrent synovial sarcoma of the right anterior chest wall. Scarring from the previous excision of the primary tumour including the medial half of the right clavicle and the anterior end of the 1st rib. Three courses of radiotherapy had been given. The skin over the tumour is red and thin; it is very vascular. Metastases are present in both lungs

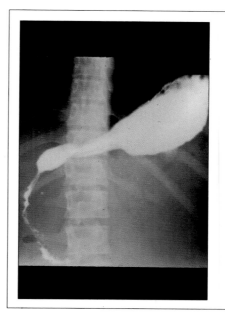

Figure 16 Radiogram with a barium meal of a male aged 26 years with a large, inoperable retroperitoneal tumour of malignant lymphoid tissue. There is marked displacement of the distal portion of the stomach and duodenum, distortion of the stomach and severe compression of the duodenum and upper jejunum

A radical excision of the fibrosarcoma was performed, removing the part of the iliac bone and separating the tumour from the peritoneum. The large defect was repaired with skin grafts. Wound healing was satisfactory and he walked well. He returned to his own country.

LIPOSARCOMA

A liposarcoma may arise in a benign lipoma, but usually it occurs *de novo*. A large lipoma may become malignant, especially when it is not completely excised. Figures 11 and 12 show a patient who was referred with an enormous lipoma involving the whole left side of the neck and extending upwards into the left face. This tumour was excised with a good cosmetic result.

A liposarcoma shows a predilection for the shoulder region, the thigh and the retroperitoneal regions. Figures 13 and 14 show a patient with a large retroperitoneal liposarcoma.

A radical resection of this tumour was carried out.

SYNOVIAL SARCOMA

Synovial sarcomas develop from synovial membrane and are usually found in the extremities, more frequently in the lower than in the upper, and connected with the foot or knee. Some of these tumours develop apart from actual synovial membrane. These tumours vary in size, are circumscribed or diffuse and are firm in consistency, but those which are rapidly-growing are soft and may be friable. Cysts may be present containing straw coloured or blood stained fluid. Necrosis and areas of haemorrhage may occur. Metastases occur in the lungs and bones in addition to lymph nodes. Recurrence may follow resection of the tumour.

Case record A female aged 55 years presented with a large recurrent tumour in the right upper chest wall following a previous surgical excision in another country.

Examination showed a curved scar 10 cm long over the anterior aspect of the right upper chest wall. There was induration at the root of the right neck, but no enlarged lymph nodes. A large tumour of the anterior chest wall measuring 8.5 cm long was pushing the chest forward on the right upper aspect (Figure 15). The tumour retained some mobility and was elastic in consistency, and the overlying skin was thin, red and hot. There were no enlarged right axillary lymph nodes. The right biceps muscle was paralysed and movements at the right shoulder joint were restricted. The volume in the right radial pulse was much diminished.

The chest radiogram showed that the medial half of the right clavicle and the anterior end of the first right rib had been excised. There was a large oval mass, presumably situated in the right upper lobe of the lung. Several metastases were present in the middle and lower zones of the right lung, and several were present in the left lung.

Histopathology sections of the primary tumour showed a typical synovial sarcoma featuring the characteristic 'biphasic' pattern, with spindle cell growth, together with gland-like spaces containing mucin. There was moderate mitotic activity.

Three aspirations of the recurrent tumour were carried out and almost pure blood was removed. The tension in the overlying skin of the tumour was thereby diminished and it was felt that these measures would continue to avoid skin ulceration if possible.

The tumour was considered to be inoperable and three courses of radiotherapy had also been given so that this was now contraindicated. Chemotherapy was given without any tumour response.

MALIGNANT LYMPHOID TISSUE TUMOUR

Case record A male aged 26 years had noticed that for 2 months his upper abdomen had become prominent and hard. He had constant pain and vomiting after each meal. He experienced anorexia and constipation with weight loss. A prominent hard tumour was found which was symmetrical around the umbilicus, smooth, lobulated, and measured 25 × 20 cm. An X-ray with a barium meal showed marked displacement of the distal portion of the stomach and duodenum with distortion of the stomach and severe compression of the duodenum and upper jejunum (Figure 16). An exploratory laparotomy was performed and a large retroperitoneal tumour was found involving the whole posterior abdominal wall, extending into the mesentery and causing pressure on the adjacent small intestine. There were no dilated loops of bowel. On biopsy, histopathology showed the appearances of a malignant lymphoid tissue tumour.

The tumour was inoperable. A short course of radiotherapy was given which was not well tolerated, and this was followed by chemotherapy. The abdominal tumour regressed considerably in size and the patient's general condition improved. He returned to his own country to continue chemotherapy.

19

Malignant melanoma

Malignant melanoma is a highly virulent tumour which occurs both in animals and humans. In animals, dogs are most often affected and the tumour is usually found in the skin. Rarely the mucous membrane of the mouth is the site. In humans, the disease may occur at any age, but there is a greater frequency from the fifth decade onwards. The commonest site affected is the skin, especially of the lower extremity, and other important sites are the skin of the head and neck, face and trunk. Attention is also directed to malignant melanoma of various parts of the eye, of the mucous membrane of the mouth and oesophagus, and of the ano-rectal region and vulva. The author has been particularly interested in malignant melanoma for many years and was a member of a small group which met in New York, USA to decide the present nomenclature of malignant melanoma. The references include two of his publications on this subject[1,2].

METASTASIZING POTENTIAL

The facility possessed by malignant tumours to reproduce themselves in other organs and tissues varies according to their cell type. The malignant melanoma has a high metastasizing potential and metastases may appear almost simultaneously with the primary tumour, which may be very small. This property depends upon certain characteristic features of the malignant melanoblast, its type cell contrasting with the cells of other tumours which possess a low metastasizing potential, such as the basal cell carcinoma. The latter type is composed of a mass of cells which are closely adherent to each other and do not tend to separate into individual units. In contrast, the malignant melanoblast is an individual unit possessing a greater degree of cell autonomy than the cells of other malignant tumours. It is therefore possible for a single malignant melanoblast to survive and produce a new colony of cells, and it will survive in the environment of highly specialized tissues.

Another feature is the tendency of malignant melanoblasts to separate from the main tumour and be carried away in the blood- or lymphatic streams to commence a new tumour colony in another locality. The chance of an active, single, malignant melanoblast becoming detached from its parent tumour is high. The single cell is able to pass through the larger lymphatic vessels and becomes arrested in the fine filtering system in the liver, lung, or bone marrow. The filtering system in these organs is similar to a virus filter. On the other hand, when a cluster of malignant melanoblasts are detached they are arrested in the regional lymph nodes.

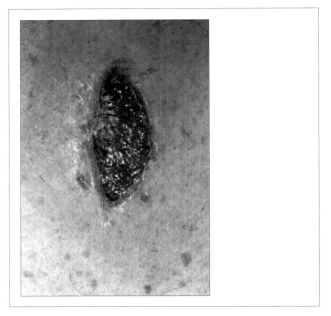

Figure 1 Malignant melanoma of the skin of the back — reddish in colour with surrounding small similar tumours

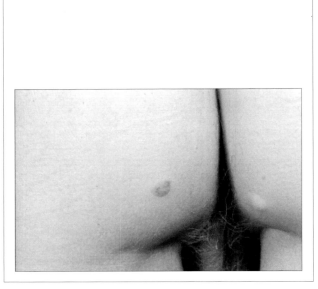

Figure 2 Malignant melanoma of the skin of the left buttock; a small reddish tumour

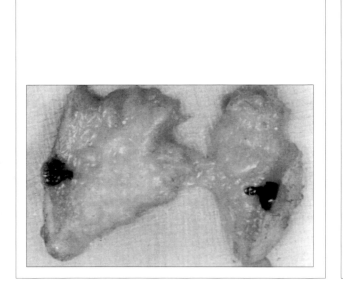

Figure 3 Malignant melanoma of the skin of the buttock showing the black tumour widely excised; note the penetration of the tumour into the subcutaneous fat

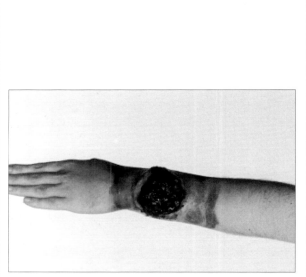

Figure 4 Malignant melanoma of the skin of the posterior aspect of the forearm

CLINICAL FEATURES OF MALIGNANT MELANOMA

The skin

The tumour is usually round and raised from the surface, to which it is attached by a broad base. The colour varies from pale and amelanotic to deep red or black. The surface is moist and superficial ulceration is often present. The consistency is firm and sometimes smaller tumours are arranged around the circumference of the main lesion. The regional lymph nodes may be enlarged and there may be small deposits of tumour along the lymphatic vessels. Sometimes the primary tumour is flat and more diffuse.

In the subungual variety the tumour projects from beneath the nail-bed, or a black halo is seen around the nail-bed. It was pointed out by Jonathan Hutchinson (1828–1913)[3] long ago that this variety of malignant melanoma has a favourable prognosis.

Figures 1–11 are illustrations of different skin malignant melanomas.

Malignant melanoma of the eye

Malignant melanoma of the eye and orbit is a rare tumour; the majority of these tumours occur between the ages of 40 and 60 years and about equally in males and in females. The tumour extends locally to involve the orbital tissues. Dissemination occurs through the bloodstream to form distant metastases, especially in the liver.

The typical malignant melanoma arises in the outer layers of the choroid and spreads locally in the eye, causing detachment of the retina and gradually filling the eye with tumour. The tumour eventually infiltrates into the orbital tissues, or presents in the anterior part of the eye. Figures 12–15 illustrate malignant melanoma of the eye.

Malignant melanoma of the oesophagus

Primary malignant melanoma is a very rare tumour in the oesophagus. A case report published by Raven and Dawson[4] and outlined in Chapter 5 is repeated here for completeness. The authors described the pathological and clinical features and tabulated the cases reported in the literature up to that date (1964). They pointed out that the presence of melanoblasts in the oesophageal epithelium provides the basic reason for the occurrence of malignant melanoma in the oesophagus. In their patient, melanin-containing cells were found in the junctional epithelium adjacent to the tumour. The reason is not known why melanoblasts are found in this situation; they may migrate there from the neural crest, or are formed by differentiation of the basal cells.

Case record   A female aged 52 years had for several months experienced discomfort across the anterior chest and lower dorsal region of the back when eating food, so that she became afraid to eat. She experienced no dysphagia, but had soreness in the upper epigastrium. She had the sensation of 'something like a lump of cotton wool' in her gullet and excessive salivation. She had no nausea, vomiting or food regurgitation and her symptoms were inconstant, so that sometimes she felt well. Investigations included radiology (Figure 16) and oesophagoscopy.

Oesophagoscopy revealed a tumour causing oesophageal rigidity, situated 25 cm from the incisor teeth with marked dilatation above it. A biopsy was performed; histopathology showed an anaplastic, very cellular carcinoma.

A partial oesophago-gastrectomy was performed through a right thoracotomy with an oesophago-gastric anastomosis, after preliminary mobilization of the stomach. On palpation of the oesophagus two tumours were felt; there was no evidence of direct spread or intrathoracic metastases.

The patient made an uninterrupted recovery and was well for 5 months. She died $13\frac{1}{2}$ months after the operation with disseminated malignant melanoma.

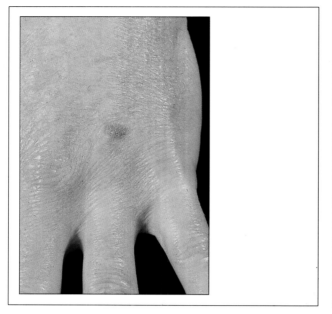

Figure 5 Malignant melanoma of the skin of the back of the hand

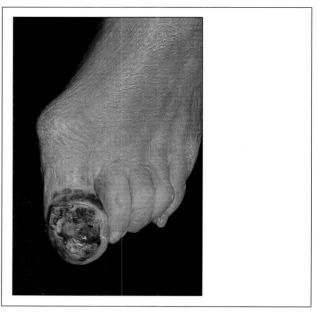

Figure 6 Malignant melanoma of the left big toe

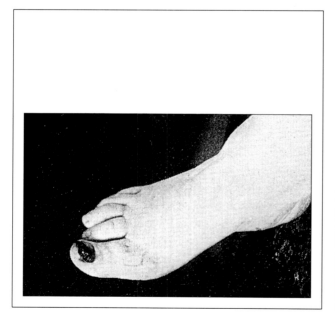

Figure 7 Malignant melanoma of the base of the big toe

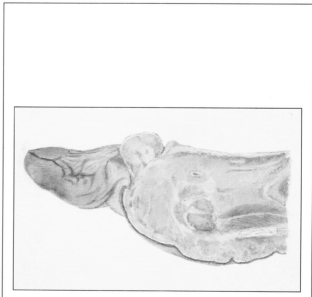

Figure 8 Subungual malignant melanoma of a big toe

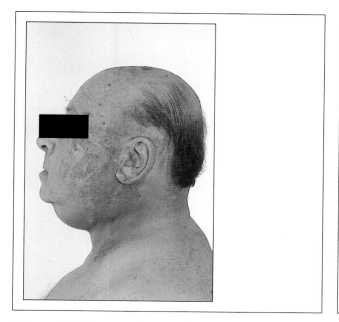

Figure 9 Malignant melanoma of the skin of the left side of the face

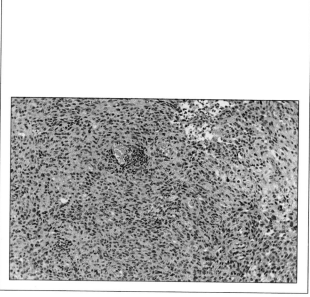

Figure 10 Histopathology study of malignant melanoma showing undifferentiated melanoma cells arranged in an alveolar pattern. A number of cells have become detached from each other and these detached cells lie in clear spaces (H & E)

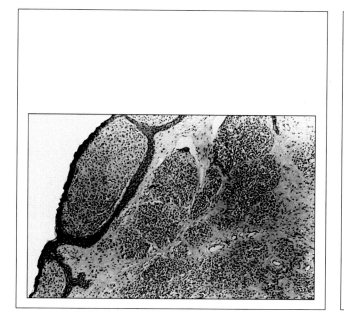

Figure 11 Histopathology study of a melanotic naevus showing the typical grouping of naevus cells in the dermis and the pseudo-intraepidermal arrangement of a compound naevus. This lesion is premalignant

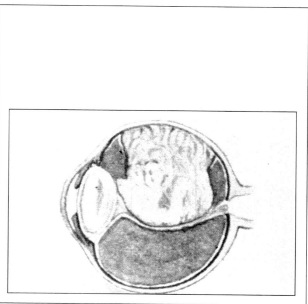

Figure 12 Malignant melanoma of the eye affecting the choroid

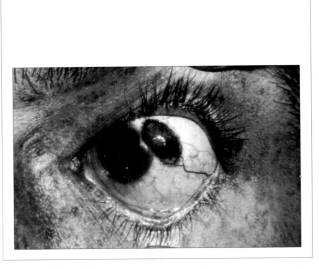

Figure 13 Malignant melanoma of the eye presenting anteriorly

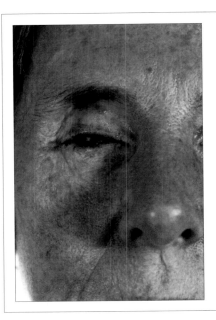

Figure 14 Malignant melanoma of the right eye affecting the orbital tissues and disseminating

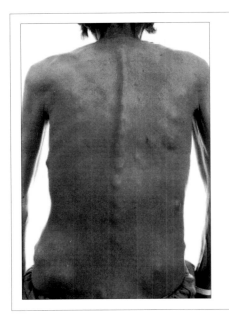

Figure 15 Malignant melanoma of the right eye disseminating to form multiple skin metastases in the back

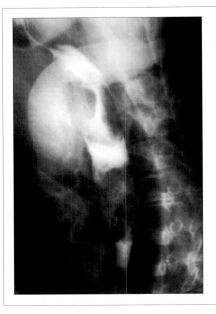

Figure 16 Radiograph of oesophagus with a barium swallow. This shows a tumour of the oesophagus involving approximately 7.5 cm in the upper limit and 12.5 cm in the lower limit. The tumour is situated about 5 cm above the cardio-oesophageal orifice; there is a small amount of barium above the tumour

The tumour specimen consisted of the distal 12 cm of oesophagus, the cardio-oesophageal junction and a ring of gastric tissue approximately 2 cm wide. In the upper part of the oesophagus was a non-pigmented polypoid tumour arising from a broad circular base 1.5 cm in diameter. Immediately below the tumour the oesophageal lumen was constricted; distal to this constriction and 1.5 cm from the upper tumour was a second large non-pigmented, flat, ulcerated tumour, which was neither polypoid nor pedunculated. It extended downwards for 5 cm almost to the cardio-oesophageal junction and occupied three-quarters of the oesophageal circumference, markedly narrowing the lumen. The mucosa around the upper tumour, and between the two tumours, and the narrow strip which remained uninvolved by the lower tumour, all appeared normal and showed no obvious pigmentation.

Blocks were taken from both tumours, from the oesophageal epithelium adjacent to both tumours and from the intervening mucosa. Sections from each block were stained with haematoxylin and eosin. Masson-Fontana silver impregnation technique and Schmorl's technique with neutral red counterstain were used to identify melanin pigment. Hydrogen peroxide was used as a bleaching agent.

The upper polypoid tumour consisted of sheets of irregularly-shaped pleomorphic cells arranged without pattern; tumour giant cells with multiple nuclei and cells in mitosis were moderately frequent. There was a clearly visible origin from the basal layer of oesophageal mucosa which showed conspicuous junctional change such as is seen in malignant melanoma and junctional naevi in the skin. The tumour was confined to the muscularis mucosae and had not invaded the submucosa or muscle coats; its clear origin from the epithelium proved it was not a metastasis. The majority of its cells were non-pigmented, but occasional tumour cells containing melanin pigment were present in it.

The lower tumour showed a similar general histopathology appearance with tumour cells containing melanin pigment present. It appeared to have originated in the submucosa and had ulcerated through the overlying epithelium, which was attenuated and did not show any junctional change, and had grown down into the muscle coats. The appearances suggested a secondary deposit from the upper tumour and this was borne out by the finding of submucosal islands of tumour between the two tumours.

The epithelium in the immediate vicinity of the upper pedunculated tumour also showed extensive junctional changes. There were isolated small zones of junctional change between the two tumours, but none below the upper limits of the lower tumour.

Melanin-containing cells resembling the melanoblasts and melanophores of the skin were present in these junctional zones, and there were very occasional similar cells in the epithelium of the upper and lower oesophagus which did not show junctional change.

Malignant melanoma of the ano-rectal region

Malignant melanoma in the ano-rectal region is a relatively uncommon tumour. The tumour arises in the skin of the anal canal or at the anal verge, and the rectum may be involved by direct extension. It very rarely develops primarily in the rectum. The posterior wall of the anal canal is the usual site, followed by the lateral walls; involvement of the anterior wall is the most infrequent site.

Varieties of tumour

A single tumour is formed usually, but a smaller tumour may be present, the two separated by apparently normal tissue. In some patients there may be a small anal tumour with a larger tumour in the ampulla of the rectum, or the primary tumour may be surrounded by a number of small satellites. The size

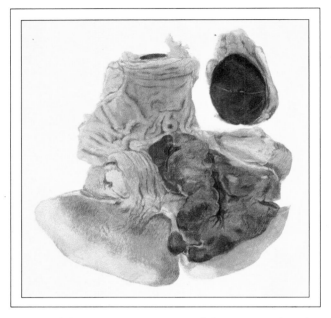

Figure 17 Malignant melanoma of the ano-rectal region with a lymph node metastasis

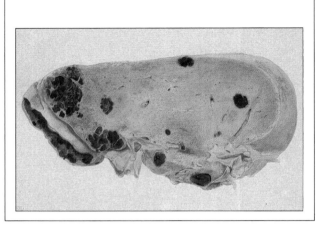

Figure 18 Malignant melanoma metastases in the liver

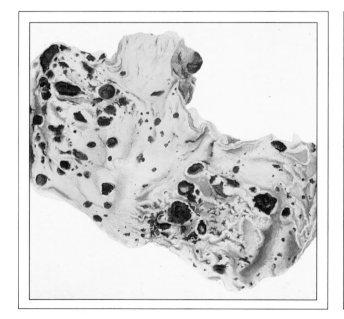

Figure 19 Malignant melanoma metastases in the stomach – multiple black tumours

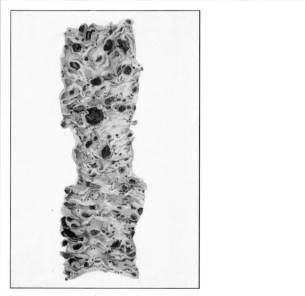

Figure 20 Malignant melanoma metastases in the small intestine – multiple black tumours

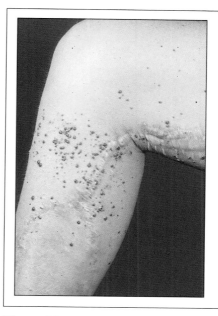

Figure 22 Malignant melanoma metastases in skin of right lower extremity. Patient had an excision of a malignant melanoma of the skin of right leg with removal of fascial strip to groin and an ilio-inguinal lymph node block dissection. Multiple skin metastatic malignant melanoma tumours occurred. Treatment with right external iliac regional perfusion with melphalan caused temporary improvement

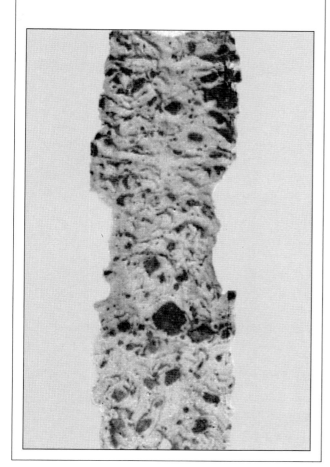

Figure 21 Malignant melanoma metastases in the colon – multiple small black tumours

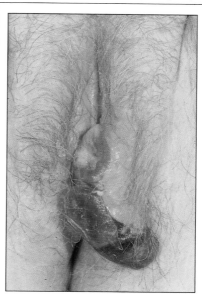

Figure 23 Primary malignant melanoma of the vulva. The tumour is pigmented and spreading from the labia

varies from a miliary nodule to a large tumour, with many intermediate varieties. The tumours may be sessile or pedunculated. In this region it is characteristic for the tumour to become pedunculated and prolapse through the anal orifice. Its base is often mobile over the deeper tissues; the surface is lobulated and areas of superficial ulceration are present. The tumour is usually black with melanin, but may be amelanotic and its consistency is firm and elastic or sometimes it feels fluctuant.

Spread of the tumour

By direct extension   There is a marked tendency for the tumour to spread from the anal canal to the rectum along the submucous tissues. Spread also occurs laterally into the tissues around the anus and rectum, but this seems to be delayed by the fascia propria of the rectum. Surrounding structures including the urinary bladder, uterus, vagina and sacrum are not usually invaded, in contradistinction to adenocarcinoma. Outlying tumour nodules may be found in the ischiorectal fossa or in the cellular tissues in the hollow of the sacrum.

Lymphatic spread   The ilio-inguinal lymph nodes are frequently involved by metastases. In cases where one lateral wall of the anal canal is affected, only the lymph nodes on the same side may be involved. A mild form of lymphadenitis may be present without metastases. When the rectum is infiltrated by the tumour, its lymphatics are also involved, as in adenocarcinoma. Lymph node metastases are usually black, even if the primary tumour is amelanotic. Involvement of the lymphatic system may be more generalized, including the thoracic duct, mesenteric, mediastinal and cervical groups of lymph nodes.

Figure 17 shows a malignant melanoma of the anorectal region with a lymph node metastasis.

Haematogenous spread   Invasion of the blood vessels causes widespread metastases, but they may be delayed for several years. The liver is frequently affected and becomes large due to nodules which may be black or amelanotic. The peritoneum may be studded with neoplastic nodules, which may also be present in the small intestine, greater omentum and appendices epiploicae. The lungs and pleura are involved frequently, and also the subcutaneous tissues, kidney, brain and meninges, pancreas, spleen, thyroid and skeleton are other sites for metastases.

METASTASES OF MALIGNANT MELANOMA

Metastases of malignant melanoma are common in the liver and are usually multiple and black (Figure 18). Malignant melanoma does not metastasize to the gastro-intestinal canal with any frequency; Figures 19–22 are therefore of interest.

PRIMARY MALIGNANT MELANOMA OF THE VULVA

Primary malignant melanoma is a rare tumour of the vulva. It develops usually in the labium majus and occasionally in the labium minus. The tumour is a raised swelling in the labium with a smooth surface; sometimes it is pedunculated. It is usually pigmented and black in colour and ulceration occurs, causing bleeding (Figure 23).

Spread of the tumour

The tumour spreads by direct extension into the surrounding tissues. Spread also occurs by the lymphatics to form metastases in the regional lymph nodes in the groin. Haematogenous metastases also develop in distant organs and tissues as with other varieties of malignant melanoma.

REFERENCES

1. Raven, R. W. (1950). The properties and surgical problems of malignant melanoma (Hunterian lecture). Delivered at the Royal College of Surgeons of England, 7 February, 1949. *Ann. R. Coll. Surg. of England*, **6**, 28–55
2. Raven, R. W. (1953). Problems concerning melanoma in man. In *Pigment Cell Growth*. (New York, N.Y.: Academic Press, Inc.)
3. Raven, R. W. and Dawson, I. (1964). Malignant melanoma of the oesophagus. *Br. J. Surg.*, **51**, pp. 551–5

20

Argentaffinoma tumours

The argentaffinoma is a very interesting tumour and it is somewhat rare when compared with the incidence of other tumours. The tumour secretes chemical substances which cause systemic metabolic disturbances, recognized as the 'argentaffinoma syndrome'. Wakeley[1] stated that the term 'carcinoid tumour' was introduced first by Oberndorfer in 1907 and the term 'karzinoid' was used until the early 1930s for small tumours in the vermiform appendix and the small intestine. Wakeley also stated that the term 'argentaffin' was introduced by Gosset and Masson in 1914 because these tumours were proved to arise from the specialized epithelial cells of Kultschitzky.

The argentaffinoma usually occurs in the gastrointestinal tract, frequently in the appendix and it has a predilection for the terminal ileum. It is found also in the stomach, duodenum, large intestine and rectum. The tumour also occurs in other sites including the bronchus, gall bladder, mesentery and Meckel's diverticulum. It is interesting that argentaffinomas have been found in ovarian teratomas, connected with the gastrointestinal and respiratory tissues in those tumours.

ARGENTAFFINOMA SYNDROME

Patients with this syndrome manifest the pharmacological effects of the excessive production by the argentaffinoma of serotonin, killikrein, and other proteolytic enzymes. The symptomatology varies somewhat according to the site of the argentaffinoma, but the outstanding feature is the cyanotic skin flushes which accompany the other symptoms. When the tumour occurs in the lower intestinal tract there are abdominal cramps, watery diarrhoea and bronchospasm. Stenotic lesions develop in the right side of the heart. When the tumour occurs elsewhere, including the bronchus, the symptomatology is somewhat different and includes facial oedema, salivation, lacrimation, tachycardia, tremor, fever, anxiety, depression, and stenotic lesions in the left side of the heart and bronchioectasis.

Treatment

The treatment of patients with this syndrome is excision, if possible, of the region containing the argentaffinoma which is secreting the serotonin. There are special risks involved in these operations. During anaesthesia severe bronchospasm or hypotension may develop, necessitating the administration of anti-serotonin drugs. When the terminal ileum is resected, the local circulation of serotonin causes vasospasm of the mesenteric blood vessels, requiring the removal of a longer segment of intestine to ensure an adequate blood supply to the anastomotic site.

During the postoperative period there may be severe abdominal pain with rigidity of the abdominal

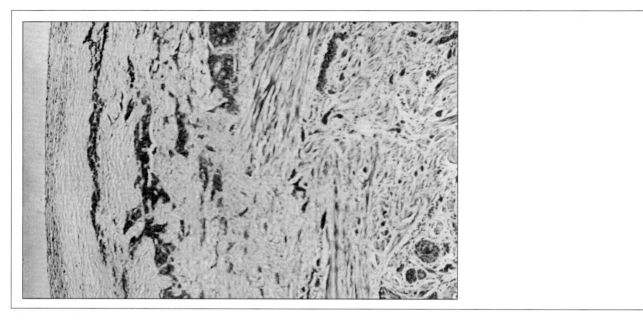

Figure 1 Histopathology of argentaffinoma of the vermi-form appendix (H & E)

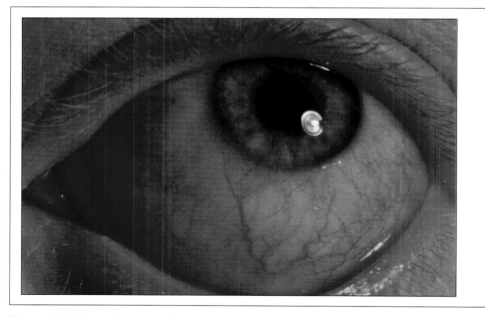

Figure 2 Patient with argentaffinoma metastases in the liver showing redness of the conjunctiva

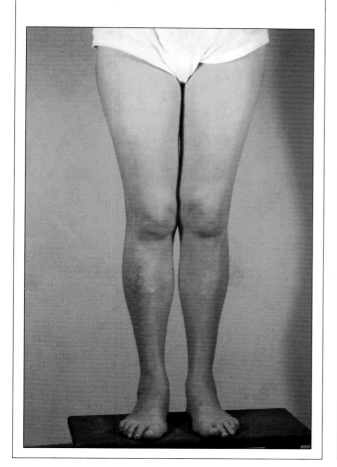

Figure 3 Patient with argentaffinoma metastases in the liver showing flushing of the skin of the lower extremities

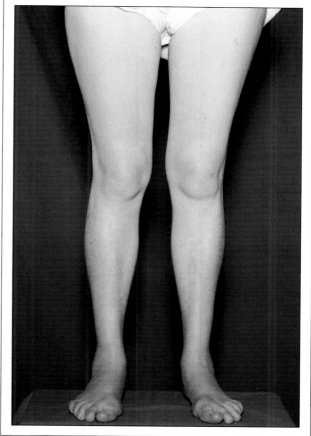

Figure 4 Patient with argentaffinoma metastases in the liver showing skin of lower extremities after flushing

wall, but without ileus; the abdomen should not be opened for this condition.

Case record A patient had a carcinoma of the lower end of the oesophagus and the cardiac portion of the stomach which infiltrated the left lobe of the liver. The whole tumour was removed surgically. Histopathology of the excised tumour confirmed the carcinoma, but in the portion of the excised liver there was a metastatic nodule of argentaffinoma. Subsequently a laparotomy was performed and two primary argentaffinomas, a metastatic lymph node and several metastases in the right lobe of the liver were found; a partial enterectomy, right hemicolectomy and partial right hepatectomy were performed.

ARGENTAFFINOMA OF THE APPENDIX

An argentaffinoma of the vermiform appendix is a small yellow tumour which is found at or near the tip. Histopathology showed that these tumours have invasive properties, but they cause local symptomatology including appendicular colic, so are removed early before any spread of the disease occurs (Figure 1).

ARGENTAFFINOMA OF THE RECTUM

This subject was reviewed by the author[2], who described three main groups of clinical cases: (1) asymptomatic cases, when the tumour is discovered at examination of the rectum for another condition such as fissure or haemorrhoids, or in a rectum excised for carcinoma; (2) metastatic cases, when the patient presents with symptoms caused by metastases of argentaffinoma in other organs, especially the liver, the primary tumour being silent; and (3) cases with rectal symptoms including bleeding, either bright or dark red in colour, a change in bowel habit with increasing constipation, diarrhoea and tenesmus. The

tumour may be single and usually occurs in the anterior rectal wall; it may be completely submucosal, or there is a partial covering of mucous membrane. It is freely mobile unless infiltration has developed. The type is variable so that a nodule, polyp, plaque, or an annular constriction may be felt, and in some patients the size may equal any malignant rectal tumour. The consistency is rubbery or firm and in some patients there is infiltration of adjacent tissues; the colour varies from white or yellow to red-brown. The rectal argentaffinoma is capable of causing widespread metastases. The distribution of metastases resembles that seen in bowel adenocarcinoma; the liver and regional lymph nodes are most often involved. Metastases are described in other organs, including kidneys, suprarenal glands, spleen, brain, lungs, bone, subcutaneous tissues and mediastinal lymph nodes.

The following treatment programme was advised by Raven[2]. When an argentaffinoma has been excised in the belief that it was an adenomatous polyp, but subsequent histopathology proves its true nature, the patient is kept under observation to detect any recurrence. When a small non-infiltrating argentaffinoma is found and confirmed by biopsy, a wide local excision is performed and the patient kept under observation. A radical operation is performed when a large argentaffinoma with infiltrating properties, or an annular constricting argentaffinoma is present. If a recurrent argentaffinoma appears, a radical operation is done.

Case record A female patient aged 60 years complained of continuous pain in the rectum and tenesmus. There was no bleeding or diarrhoea; she had suffered from constipation for many years. On rectal examination there was a firm polyp arising from the right lateral wall, 3 cm from the anus. Large internal haemorrhoids were also present and sigmoidoscopy showed no other abnormality up to 20 cm from the anal orifice. A haemorrhoidectomy and excision of the polyp were performed. Histopathology appearances of the polyp were those of an argentaffinoma.

The patient is well and had no sign of recurrence 6 months later.

ARGENTAFFINOMA HEPATIC METASTASES

When argentaffinoma metastases do occur, the liver is the most common site and these patients present important problems in their management[3]. The following case is that of a patient who was referred with hepatic argentaffinoma metastases 31 years ago.

Case record A female aged 32 years was investigated for severe skin flushes which occurred intermittently in the face, and upper and lower extremities, accompanied by redness of the conjunctiva. Investigations showed normal haematology; alkaline phosphatase was 6 units/100 ml; bilirubin was 0.7 mg/100 ml; albumin was 4.2 mg/100 ml; globulin was 3.9 mg/100 ml; liver function tests showed the albumin : globulin ratio to be 1.1 : 1, and the serum protein electrophoresis showed the gamma globulin to be slightly prominent. The 5-hydroxy indole acetic acid (HIAA) excretion was 114 mg in 24 h (normal 2–8 mg in 24 h). Radiological examination of the gastrointestinal tract with a barium meal showed very rapid passage of the barium through the small and large intestines, so that the head of the meal had reached the rectum by 2 h and the small intestine was not clearly outlined.

An exploratory laparotomy revealed multiple small argentaffinoma metastases in both lobes of the liver, varying in size from a pinpoint to 1 cm in diameter. A Meckel's diverticulum was present in the ileum and above this a nodule was felt in the ileum about the size of a split pea; another nodule 12.5 cm proximal to it and about 1.25 cm in diameter was invading the bowel muscular coat; an enlarged lymph node was present nearby in the mesentery. A partial enterectomy of about 25 cm was carried out, removing the nodules and adjacent mesentery with the enlarged lymph node. An end-to-end enteric anastomasis was done, as well as a liver biopsy. During the operation considerable intestinal peristalsis was noted.

The patient made a good recovery. The postoperative 5-HIAA excretion was 41 mg in 24 h.

Histopathology showed the various nodules from the ileum and liver to have islands of polygonal cells of variable size, with lightly staining nuclei and cytoplasm containing argyrophilic granules. The fibrous stroma was variable, being most dense in the hepatic nodule. In the larger ileal nodule, infiltration had occurred through the wall to the peritoneum. The appearances were those of argentaffinoma of the ileum with omental and hepatic metastases.

Figures 2–4 show the typical skin flushes of the argentaffinoma syndrome as seen in this patient.

REFERENCES

1. Wakeley, Sir Cecil (1958). Argentaffinoma (carcinoid) tumours. In Raven, R. W. (ed.) *Cancer*, Vol. 4, Ch. 13, pp. 162–6. (London: Butterworth & Co. Ltd)
2. Raven, R. W. (1950). Carcinoid tumours of the rectum. *Proc. R. Soc. Med.*, **43**, 675–7
3. Raven, R. W. (1957). Liver surgery in relation to diseases of the colon and rectum. *Proc. R. Soc. Med.*, **50**, 775–86

21

Angioma and haemangiosarcoma tumours

ANGIOMA

A benign angioma is an uncommon tumour but it can be disfiguring and serious as exemplified by the patient shown in Figure 1.

HAEMANGIOSARCOMA

Malignant tumours of undoubted vascular origin are very rare. Some of the examples reported in the literature exhibited haematogenous metastases, whilst in others the primary tumour disseminated to the regional lymph nodes. The interesting case of haemangiosarcoma reported by Raven and Christie[1] showed both lymphatic and haematogenous metastases; dissemination of this tumour by both methods simultaneously is extremely rare, so a detailed account of this patient is given here.

Case record   A female aged 61 years stated that she had had an extensive naevus of the skin of her left arm since her birth. Multiple operations to remove it had been performed during childhood, the first when she was aged 2 years. A lump had developed in her left arm 5 years previously and this had been excised 6 months earlier.

Examination showed a large diffuse 'angioma' affecting the posterior aspect of the left arm, which extended from a point 5 cm below the posterior axillary fold down to the region of the wrist. Its extent was minimal in the forearm and maximal in the upper arm, where, on the outer aspect bordering on part of the 'angioma', there was a recurrent tumour which measured 5 × 3 cm close to one of the numerous old healed surgical scars. There was no other abnormality.

The recurrent tumour of the left arm was widely excised and included part of the sheath of the underlying triceps muscle. The tumour consisted of an irregular mass of encapsulated angiomatous tissue measuring 6 cm in its longest dimension, which extended into the deep fascia and contained areas of recent haemorrhage and thrombosis.

A further recurrent tumour was widely excised after 8 months, and another after 15 months. Both tumours were ill-defined, non-encapsulated and haemorrhagic, lying in the subcutaneous tissues and extending into the adjacent muscle. Arteriograms and phlebograms had not shown any penetration of the tumour by radio-opaque dye.

Another extensive recurrent tumour occurred later. A chest radiogram showed no metastases and an amputation of the upper limb was advised; the patient refused, so a course of radiotherapy was given to the tumour. No regression occurred in the tumour and there was no evidence of metastases so the

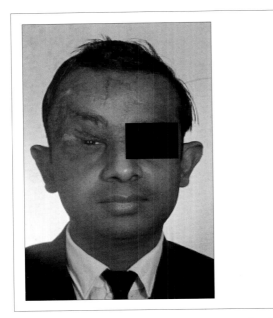

Figure I Patient with an angioma involving the right frontal region of the scalp and the right upper eyelid

patient agreed to an amputation; an interscapulo-thoracic amputation of the left upper extremity was performed. The patient was recovering well and was fully ambulant when a massive pulmonary embolism occurred 17 days following the operation and proved fatal.

A description of the amputated limb and tumour was given by the pathologist. The limb was markedly oedematous throughout and the structures of the upper arm were greatly distorted by a massive encircling tumour which, medially and posteriorly, had produced raised ulcerated areas of tumour of firm consistency up to 13 × 10 cm in size. Elsewhere the intact skin surface showed firm, bluish, projecting tumours, the largest measuring 3.5 × 3 × 1 cm, with soft, cystic, pink and blue protrusions. Scattered beyond these, almost to the wrist distally and to within 15 cm of the shoulder joint on the posterior axillary wall, were ill-defined purplish areas of cutaneous discoloration. In the subcutaneous tissue of the thoracic wall there was a separate tumour mass, 4.5 cm in its main diameter, which infiltrated the underlying muscle. The veins in the muscles between this tumour and the axillary wall, as well as in the basilic, axillary and subclavian vessels, contained dark red and whitish thrombus, both loose and adherent to the intima.

Two enlarged lymph nodes, 4.5 × 3.0 × 2.3 cm and 1.5 cm in diameter respectively, were present in the axilla; each node contained soft, dark red and partly whitish tumour metastases.

On histopathology, the recurrent haemangiosarcoma excised locally showed diffuse invasion of the fatty, subcutaneous tissue by masses of vasoformative tissue in an abundant stroma of dense, partly hyalinized, often haemorrhagic connective tissue, interspersed with numerous clefts, occasionally filled with erythrocytes, but mostly empty and lined sometimes by a single layer, but more often by irregular masses, of endothelial cells. Although in occasional places giving the appearance of a typical benign cavernous angioma, the architecture for the most part was disorderly, with invasion of the surrounding fatty tissue by masses of closely packed, long, slender spindle cells often arranged in whorled fasciculi, bearing a strong resemblance to a spindle cell sarcoma; or grouped so as to form narrow, elongated cords which, on cross-section, contained small, centrally-situated groups of two, three, or sometimes more, plump polyhedral cells with rounded, or often indented, ovoid vesicular nuclei. In formalin-fixed and paraffin-embedded sections stained with haematoxylin and eosin, the latter had a well-defined nuclear membrane and a fairly reticular chromatin pattern with a variable number of small chromatin knots at the intersection of the fine threads, but no actual nucleoli. Sometimes the cytoplasm of these rounded central cells was vacuolated with the nucleus pushed to the periphery, giving the appearance of incipient lumen formation.

Each recurrent tumour showed a similar histopathology appearance, only varying with the relative amounts of spindle cell sarcoma-like tissue and blood-containing angiomatous areas.

Histopathology from the upper arm removed by interscapulothoracic amputation showed widespread infiltration of the skin and subcutaneous tissue by well-developed capillary angiosarcoma, and sheets of anaplastic cells with pleomorphic and hyperchromatic nuclei, the latter only occasionally showing vasoformative tendencies characteristic of the previous recurrences. For the first time occasional giant cells with single bizarre nuclei were present. Mitotic figures were very rare in all recurrences. In the subcutaneous tissue small clumps of anaplastic tumour cells were invading perivascular and perineural lymphatics.

The smaller axillary lymph node was replaced by haemorrhagic tumour tissue, in some places showing a closely packed and whorled spindle cell structure, and in others a histological pattern closely resembling a cavernous angioma.

Necropsy results showed that the amputation incision was healing by first intention. The right lung, in a pleural cavity free of adhesions and excess fluid, contained three tumour metastases. Two metastases were in the upper lobe, the larger measuring 0.5 cm in diameter, and the smaller approximately 8×4 mm in cross-section; the larger caused slight bulging of the overlying pleura. The third metastasis was situated subpleurally in the lower lobe and measured 2 cm in its longest pleural dimension and 8 mm deep. It was paler and firmer than the deeply congested parenchyma.

The left lung, bound to the parietal pleura by numerous old fibrous adhesions, contained five small, deep red, firm, encapsulated metastases; three were subpleural and two were within the substance of the lobes, the larger being spherical.

Both main pulmonary arteries and their primary branches were occluded by large twisted emboli, and many of their smaller divisions by secondary thrombi, the latter having arisen *in situ*. Both lungs were deeply congested, making it difficult to detect the small metastases, which, with one exception already mentioned, were of similar dark red colour; however, they were of slightly firmer consistency than the surrounding parenchyma, thus making them easier felt than seen.

The liver, weighing 2.2 kg, contained a large, mottled red and yellowish-white, partly haemorrhagic, soft, friable, non-encapsulated metastasis, which was almost spherical and was situated in the right lobe beneath its diaphragmatic surface. It measured $9 \times 9 \times 8$ cm, and in the compressed parenchyma 2 cm away was a small, spherical, non-encapsulated, deep red metastasis 3 mm in diameter. The remainder of the liver was normal.

The deep veins of the calf of the left leg were occluded by thrombus which extended up to the popliteal fossa. The brain, thyroid gland, heart, breast, spleen, adrenal glands, kidneys and reproductive organs showed no abnormality.

The histopathology appearances in both lungs were complicated by the presence of widespread congestion, oedema, and vascular thrombosis, the latter involving both the right and left pulmonary arteries and many of their branches. Most of the metastases had a similar histology appearance. These were encapsulated expanding lesions consisting mainly of well-defined, dilated vascular spaces up to 200 μ in diameter and lined by a single layer of spindle-shaped cells, some containing phagocytosed blood pigment. However, very occasionally the vasoformative cells were grouped together in wide sheets of spindle cells showing a very poor attempt to form vascular channels but actually invading the parenchyma. At the periphery of the tumour the angiomatous tissue gave every appearance of invading the surrounding compressed parenchyma, showing a special predilection for spreading both subpleurally and perivascularly in lymphatic channels. Sometimes the tumours showed a central zone of relatively recent necrosed tissue in which the outline of thrombosed vessels and cavernous tumour tissue were still just discernible. Often in the tissues immediately surrounding these centrally necrotic deposits, both arteries and veins were compressed with obliteration of the central lumen, thus accounting for the necrosis. The small vascular tumour projecting from the surface of the left lung was a very well-organized cavernous angioma consisting of wide blood filled spaces lined by a single layer of elongated, flattened endothelial cells. The greater part of it lay outside the main pleural layer (intact throughout in this cross-section), with only a small portion within the lung. The expanding nature of the external portion was also shown. In both lungs the hilar lymph nodes were very congested, haemorrhagic, and laden with carbon-containing histiocytes, but showed no evidence of metastases.

The larger tumour in the liver contained, amidst extensive areas of thrombus, fluid blood, necrotic parenchyma, and highly cellular vasoformative tissue, in places arranged in whorls of closely packed spindle cells with densely stained, elongated nuclei, and sometimes enclosing within their meshes rounded vacuolated cells with the nucleus pushed to one side. These whorls often sent off from their periphery into the surrounding matrix of fluid blood, long narrow cords, mostly only two cells thick, of elongated endothelial cells which in places united with other cords to form cavities filled with fluid blood and gave the overall appearance of areas of cavernous angioma resembling those seen in the early metastases in the lungs. Occasionally these narrow cords enclosed strands of parenchyma, mainly only one or two cells thick, thus demonstrating a tendency of these cells to cover surfaces as well as line spaces – a property further demonstrated at the periphery of the tumour where spearheads of spindle cells were seen to penetrate, isolate, and surround cords of liver cells within the lobules. The small nearby lesion consisted of similar spindle-celled vasoformative tissue. Mitotic figures were very rare in both pulmonary and liver lesions.

A haemangioma is an extremely rare tumour in an extremity of the body; Raven and Christie[1] state that the only other example reported at that time was described by Kettle[2]. A female aged 44 years had had 'elephantiasis' of the right foot and leg since childhood and later a bluish-red discoloration of the skin developed, with attacks of sharp shooting pain. The leg was incised in several places and silk drains inserted causing temporary improvement. Later the limb was amputated through the thigh, but in less than a year the stump became hard, discoloured and very painful. This necessitated a further amputation through the hip joint, which was difficult because the tumour had extended up to the groin.

Haemangiosarcoma has been described in other sites of the body. Kettle[2] reported a female aged 4 months who developed a swelling attached to the outer border of the erector spinae muscles; Robinson and Castleman[3] reported a female aged 18 years whose right breast was affected; for this a local mastectomy was performed but recurrences developed 8 months later.

Angiosarcoma has been described in the spleen with liver metastases[4], and also in the lung causing multiple metastases[5].

The author realizes that other cases may have been reported since 1954 when he and Christie reviewed the literature and wrote their article, in which they also discussed the pathology of this rare tumour.

Pathology

Since malignant tumours of the vasoformative tissue are so rare[6] and are frequently simulated by other highly vascular malignant tumours, it was important to decide, as Raven and Christie point out, that the tumour they reported arose from vasoformative tissue. In their patient there is no doubt that the skin tumour in the left arm was a primary tumour with this origin, for much of it consisted of typical cavernous angiomatous tissue with wide sinuses filled with fluid blood and lined by a single layer of flattened endothelial cells. Other parts of the tumour closely resembled a typical spindle cell sarcoma of connective tissue with whorled masses of elongated, narrow cells, in places invading the surrounding subcutaneous tissue and the underlying muscle. Furthermore, recurrent tumours occurred fairly rapidly, and finally metastases of typical angiomatous tissue developed in the axillary lymph nodes, confirming the malignant nature of this particular tumour.

Reference is also made to the metastases in the liver and lungs in this case for it is recognized that benign angiomas can occur multifocally; it is necessary therefore to decide in each case whether the multiple tumours are metastases or hamartomas. The liver is also a common site of benign cavernous angiomas, which are usually found at autopsy. In this case the presence of a large, expanding, centrally necrotic and partly thrombosed tumour, consisting of masses of spindle cells invading the surrounding parenchyma and producing a small satellite tumour nearby, indicated that this undoubtedly was a malignant tumour. The presence of whorled spindle-celled masses throwing off cords of endothelial cells identical with that seen in parts of the primary tumour in the arm was strongly in favour of a metastasis.

Regarding the pulmonary lesions in this case, they were mostly centrally necrotic, rapidly expanding masses of cavernous angiomatous tissue which were invading the surrounding perivascular and subpleural lymphatics. These consisted of tissue resembling parts of the primary tumour and were undoubtedly metastases. It is very rare in a haemangiosarcoma to find local lymphatic spread from the primary tumour and lung metastases, in addition to distant haematogenous dissemination, as is demonstrated in this case report.

REFERENCES

1. Raven, R. W. and Christie, A. C. (1954). Haemangiosarcoma. A case with lymphatic and haematogenous metastases. *Br. J. Surg.*, **41**, 483–9
2. Kettle, E. H. (1918). Tumours arising from endothelium. *Proc. R. Soc. Med.*, **11**, 19–34
3. Robinson, J. M. and Castleman, B. (1936). Benign metastasizing hemangioma. *Ann. Surg.*, **104**, 453–9
4. Wright, A. W. (1928). Primary malignant hemangioma of spleen with multiple liver metastases. *Am. J. Pathol.*, **4**, 507–24
5. Hall, E. M. (1935). Malignant hemangioma of lung with multiple metastases. *Am. J. Pathol.*, **11**, 343–52
6. Willis, R. A. (1948). *Pathology of Tumours*, p. 704. (London: Butterworth & Co. Ltd)

Index